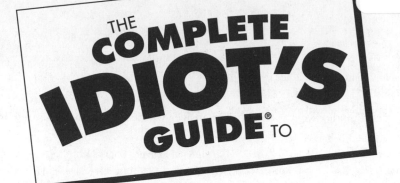

THE **COMPLETE IDIOT'S GUIDE** TO

Glycemic Index Weight Loss

by Lucy Beale and Joan Clark, M.S., R.D., C.D.E.

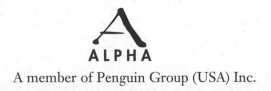

ALPHA

A member of Penguin Group (USA) Inc.

Lucy: To Patrick
Joan: To my parents, Cyril and Josephine Kinane

ALPHA BOOKS

Published by the Penguin Group

Penguin Group (USA) Inc., 375 Hudson Street, New York, New York 10014, U.S.A.

Penguin Group (Canada), 10 Alcorn Avenue, Toronto, Ontario, Canada M4V 3B2 (a division of Pearson Penguin Canada Inc.)

Penguin Books Ltd, 80 Strand, London WC2R 0RL, England

Penguin Ireland, 25 St Stephen's Green, Dublin 2, Ireland (a division of Penguin Books Ltd)

Penguin Group (Australia), 250 Camberwell Road, Camberwell, Victoria 3124, Australia (a division of Pearson Australia Group Pty Ltd)

Penguin Books India Pvt Ltd, 11 Community Centre, Panchsheel Park, New Delhi—110 017, India

Penguin Group (NZ), cnr Airborne and Rosedale Roads, Albany, Auckland 1310, New Zealand (a division of Pearson New Zealand Ltd)

Penguin Books (South Africa) (Pty) Ltd, 24 Sturdee Avenue, Rosebank, Johannesburg 2196, South Africa

Penguin Books Ltd, Registered Offices: 80 Strand, London WC2R 0RL, England

Copyright © 2005 by Lucy Beale

International Standard Book Number: 1-59257-404-1
Library of Congress Catalog Card Number: 2005923957

08 07 06   8 7 6

Interpretation of the printing code: The rightmost number of the first series of numbers is the year of the book's printing; the rightmost number of the second series of numbers is the number of the book's printing. For example, a printing code of 05-1 shows that the first printing occurred in 2005.

Printed in the United States of America

Note: This publication contains the opinions and ideas of its authors. It is intended to provide helpful and informative material on the subject matter covered. It is sold with the understanding that the authors and publisher are not engaged in rendering professional services in the book. If the reader requires personal assistance or advice, a competent professional should be consulted.

Most Alpha books are available at special quantity discounts for bulk purchases for sales promotions, premiums, fundraising, or educational use. Special books, or book excerpts, can also be created to fit specific needs.

For details, write: Special Markets, Alpha Books, 375 Hudson Street, New York, NY 10014.

Publisher: *Marie Butler-Knight*
Product Manager: *Phil Kitchel*
Senior Managing Editor: *Jennifer Bowles*
Senior Acquisitions Editor: *Renee Wilmeth*
Development Editor: *Ginny Bess Munroe*
Production Editor: *Janette Lynn*

Copy Editor: *Tricia Liebig*
Cartoonist: *Shannon Wheeler*
Cover/Book Designer: *Trina Wurst*
Indexer: *Tonya Heard*
Layout: *Angela Calvert*
Proofreading: *Donna Martin*

Contents at a Glance

Contents

Foreword

This book is the culmination of the most significant dietary advances of the past quarter century. Written with a refreshing style, this book is not only knowledgeable and balanced, but also extremely practical for millions of people.

Scientists developed the concept of the glycemic index in the 1970s. The first article in a professional journal to use that term appeared in 1981. It took many more years for consciousness of the glycemic index to seep into the general culture, and I suspect that I had something to do with that. Shortly after I received the diagnosis in February 1994 that I have diabetes, my diabetes educator mentioned that she had read an item about the glycemic index in a professional book. Somehow, that caught my attention, and I never let go of it.

But that was all I could find until April 1994 when Catherine Nord posted a message on an Internet mailing list about some foods that had been tested for the 1981 article. Her post was my breakthrough. It lead to our meeting and eventual marriage, but that's another story.

That also led to my 1996 article about the glycemic index in *Diabetes Interview* magazine, which I think was the first article anywhere about it in the popular press. Subsequently, I have written about 20 articles and co-authored one book on this subject alone and about 500 other articles on diabetes in general.

People with diabetes, like my wife and me, were among the first to appreciate the value of the glycemic index, because it helps so much in controlling our blood glucose. Then people who are trying to lose weight caught on to its significance.

People discovered that when you eat low on the glycemic index, you lower your insulin levels, increase your energy, and stop storing fat, which you begin to burn. This chain of events leads automatically to weight loss.

After one of America's largest magazines featured the weight-loss advantage of following the glycemic index in a 2003 cover story, the world at large began to know about it. That article directed readers to my website, mendosa.com, which was overwhelmed when people downloaded up to 27 billion bytes per week of my glycemic index articles.

Hundreds of people have subsequently written to thank me for helping them lose weight by avoiding high-glycemic foods. Someone even went so far as to write, "Thank God for you and your site. If angels are messengers on this earth, then you will get your wings in the next life." That seems a bit extreme, but it is true that many people are now losing weight by paying attention to the glycemic index of the food they eat.

This will work for you, too. Unlike fad diets, the glycemic index is based on science that you can follow for a lifetime. And when you pay attention to a recent extension of the glycemic index called the glycemic load, weight loss and blood glucose control becomes even easier. That's because the glycemic index tells not only how rapidly a particular carbohydrate turns into glucose, it also tells you how much of that carbohydrate is in a serving of a particular food.

You can reap great benefits from the practical use of the glycemic index and the glycemic load. Working with these concepts correctly will help you meet your goal.

—David Mendosa

Introduction

Losing weight by eating based on the glycemic index is quite simple. It will become the natural and pleasing approach you use to lose weight and get down to your ideal size, while at the same time improving your health. Dieting and deprivation will become phantoms of your past as you learn how to eat luscious, glycemic index–savvy meals that make your excess pounds melt away.

In this book, you learn why glycemic index weight loss works and how it benefits your health. This book discusses three different approaches to eating based on the glycemic index that are doable and practical. In addition, you learn about stress, insulin, and cortisol and how they interact and affect your body and weight. You also learn simple ways to turn exercise into your weight-loss friend.

If you picked up this book because you want to reach your ideal size, you are committed to succeed. With the information in this book, you can put the full force of your commitment, energy, and lifestyle in sync with your weight-loss goals. The synergy that results is sure to make you a winner of the weight-loss challenge!

How This Book Is Organized

This book is divided into seven parts:

Part 1, "All About the Glycemic Index," gives you a solid scientific and biological understanding of glycemic index weight loss. You learn how the glycemic index was first created when researchers realized that not all carbohydrates affect blood sugar and insulin levels in the same way. The glycemic index aids in weight loss, reducing insulin resistance, and boosting metabolism.

Part 2, "Designing Your Glycemic Index Weight-Loss Program," offers you a choice of two different programs, "Keep It Simple" and "Comprehensive," for attaining your weight-loss goals. You'll learn how to eat based on the new food guide pyramid and how to set goals you can meet.

Part 3, "Nutritionally Balanced Eating," shows you the value of proteins, fats, and dairy for your glycemic index weight-loss program. Learn how to deal with sugars and junk foods, plus learn important information on which nutritional supplements can enhance your weight-loss program.

Part 4, "Eating for All Occasions," gives you valuable suggestions for eating based on the glycemic index at home, at parties, and even while traveling and vacationing. You learn how to shop for groceries and how to plan low-glycemic meals.

Part 5, "Insulin, Cortisol, and Weight Loss," offers new information on the biological interactions between insulin and the stress hormone, cortisol. By keeping your stress levels low, you can enhance your weight-loss progress. We show you how.

Part 6, "The Exercise Advantage," shows you how the three types of exercise—aerobic, strength training, and stretching—all help you reduce insulin resistance and manage stress. Exercise does more than help your weight-loss efforts by burning through calories; it actually changes your biology.

Part 7, "Glycemic Index Books and Programs," reviews the popular programs and books that recommend eating based on the glycemic index. You'll find programs for health, for mid-life, and for weight loss.

Extras

We know you don't own a secret decoder ring to help you in the confusing world of glycemic index weight loss—and you shouldn't have to. This book has a few easy-to-recognize signposts that offer tips, tricks, and tidbits to help you along the way. Look for these elements in this book that will point you in the right direction:

Wrong Weigh

Watch out! Avoid these glycemic index eating pitfalls so that you don't falter, but instead gain self-confidence and self-assurance with every bite.

Glyco Lingo

With these definitions you'll be in-the-know about the science, biology, and technicalities of glycemic index weight loss.

Thin-spiration

Use these helpful tips and hints as your personal coach for achieving your weight-loss goals.

Body of Knowledge

Gain the knowledge and dietary background about glycemic index eating you need so that you can better master your eating and your weight.

Acknowledgments

Lucy and Joan give special thanks to their clients, without whom they wouldn't have gleaned the special hands-on information and practical suggestions that are added into every page of this book.

Lucy Beale thanks her husband, Patrick, for his patience and support while she was occupied and preoccupied with writing and for his valuable editing suggestions. She also thanks Pat Jr. for timely editing assistance. Lucy thanks her co-author, Joan, for her thoughtful, scientific expertise, as well as her insightful comments and suggestions.

Joan Clark thanks her children, Jenny, Ryan, and Tricia, for their patience and encouragement. Joan thanks the author, Lucy, for her expertise, enthusiasm, and creativity. She also thanks Dr. Dana Clarke for sharing his expertise on low-glycemic eating and the low-glycemic food guide pyramid.

Lucy and Joan both thank Marilyn Allen of the Allen O'Shea Literary Agency and Renee Wilmeth, senior acquisitions editor at Alpha Books, for guiding this book from inception through publication. Special thanks to Jennie Brand-Miller for permission to excerpt the glycemic index from her book, *What Makes My Blood Glucose Go Up … And Down?* written with Kaye Foster-Powell and Rick Mendosa. And to Rick Mendosa for being available to answer our questions and for creating www.mendosa.com, which offers valuable and practical information on the glycemic index.

Trademarks

All terms mentioned in this book that are known to be or are suspected of being trademarks or service marks have been appropriately capitalized. Alpha Books and Penguin Group (USA) Inc. cannot attest to the accuracy of this information. Use of a term in this book should not be regarded as affecting the validity of any trademark or service mark.

Part 1

All About the Glycemic Index

Glycemic index weight loss has never been a "fad," and for good reason. It's a highly regarded and scientifically validated method for significant and successful weight loss, as well as a way to eat to improve health and reduce the risk of chronic health conditions. Glycemic index weight loss lowers insulin levels and insulin resistance, increases energy, and even lowers stress. As your body stops storing fat, you begin to burn fat for energy while you boost your metabolism. Thus you lose weight. The glycemic index used hand-in-hand with the glycemic load will have you eating plenty of healthy, nutrient-dense carbohydrates—especially ones containing phytonutrients, antioxidants, vitamins, minerals, and dietary fiber.

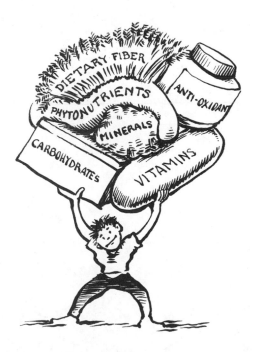

The Glycemic Index: An Amazing Weight-Loss Tool

In This Chapter

- Appreciating how the glycemic index is different
- Managing blood sugar levels
- Learning scientific research studies
- Accepting the glycemic index worldwide

If you've heard of the glycemic index, you may have already begun to use it as a guide for eating and for weight loss. Good for you. If you haven't heard about it, you're in for a treat—and not just the kind of treat you eat. Instead, it's the kind of treat that makes losing weight easy and knowing what to eat fail-proof.

The glycemic index is just plain brilliant because it's based on the science of how foods, specifically carbohydrates, work in your body. But the glycemic index isn't merely someone's good idea or an interesting intellectual theory. The glycemic index has been research-tested on real people who have the same kinds of weight-loss and health issues as you. That's how we know it works.

Beyond Other Diets

Glycemic index weight loss goes beyond any diet program you've ever tried and does what all the other programs have tried to do. For starters, it explains why you've gained weight from both biological and behavioral points of view. It teaches you how to eat adequate amounts of healthy food. It keeps your body from storing new fat by keeping your *blood sugar levels* and *insulin levels* healthy. It even lets you eat treat foods from time to time without gaining weight.

Glyco Lingo

Blood sugar levels are considered healthy when the fasting level is between 70 and 120. **Healthy insulin levels** are between 4 and 27. To find your blood glucose or your insulin levels, check with your physician. **Insulin resistance** occurs when there is a decrease in the ability of the body's cells to readily uptake glucose for energy. In other words, insulin can no longer effectively transport glucose into the cells. This condition can occur more readily when one is overweight and as one ages. In addition, some individuals may have more insulin resistance due to their genetic makeup.

Perhaps you've tried some of the diets listed next. Here's why they don't work long-term:

◆ Strict low-carbohydrate diets. They encourage you to eat large quantities of meats and fats, while limiting vegetables and fruits. Overeating all by itself encourages *insulin resistance*, which leads to weight gain.

◆ Extreme low-fat diets. Your body needs between 20 and 30 percent fat intake per day to maintain good health. This is considered low fat, but it is not extreme, and it will allow one to get adequate amounts of the essential fatty acids. Without adequate fat, your body can't release stored fat. Plus, these diets encourage us to gobble lots of low-fat, processed foods that are high in carbohydrates. Eating them can lead to insulin resistance and weight gain.

◆ Extremely low-calorie diets. Because they ignore the balance of what you need, they can be unhealthy. A person might stay within the limited calorie restrictions by eating too many high-glycemic foods, and the results will be disappointing. Calories do need to be restricted for weight loss, but it is not healthy to eat less than 1200 calories a day. This is about the minimum amount of calories needed to obtain adequate amounts of nutrients needed by the body. Indirectly, a low-calorie diet can lead to insulin resistance and weight gain.

◆ Fad diets. Diets such as the cabbage-soup diet, the liquid diet, or food combining, aren't based on scientific research and biological studies. As such, they don't offer safe and reliable long-term weight loss. Plus, they don't offer a reasonable approach to lifelong healthy eating.

> ### Body of Knowledge
>
> Is the glycemic index just another fad? The answer is a resounding No! It's a medically sound, scientifically tested explanation for how the body reacts to the foods we eat. Although we still have much to learn, the glycemic index has been researched since the 1980s and is used by nutritionists around the world to guide people—especially those with eating challenges, such as persons with diabetes.

Glycemic index weight loss keeps you out of insulin resistance, allowing you to lose weight steadily and safely while eating plenty of food. You definitely won't go hungry while following a glycemic index weight-loss program. In all fairness we should mention that you won't be eating stacks of donuts, muffins, or bagels any more. You can, however, eat them sometimes. Besides, you probably weren't eating them—except on the sly—on any other program either.

Glycemic Index for You

With this book in your hand, you have the power to lose weight safely and assuredly. Plus, the glycemic index can improve your overall health, maintain or increase lean muscle mass, and balance your moods.

That's a big claim for anything, let alone something as fundamentally simple as the glycemic index. But you'll soon understand why it's true. The basic simplicity of it is one if its strengths.

Using the glycemic index picks up where other diet programs end. Strict low-carbohydrate diet programs tend to leave you hungry and feeling deprived, which makes them hard to maintain in the long-term. Other programs that require restricting calories, drinking meal replacement shakes, and eating prepackaged meals tend to leave you feeling that "eating's no fun anymore." That's not good.

Before we tell you exactly what using the glycemic index is all about, first let us tell you what it's not:

♦ It's not a starvation program. You'll be able to eat plenty of food throughout the day and not end up ravenous in the late afternoon. You'll eat carbohydrates, fats, and proteins.

♦ It doesn't include diet phases. You won't need to endure a two-week induction phase or a special maintenance phase. The same program you start with is the one you will continue to use throughout your life.

♦ It doesn't include special diet foods. You won't need to purchase contrived specialty diet foods. Instead, you'll eat wholesome, commonly available foods. You could end up making a couple trips to the health-food store for some whole grains or sweeteners, but most of your food supply can come from your neighborhood grocery store.

♦ It doesn't contain artificial foods. You won't need to use any controversial foods, such as aspartame or highly processed packaged foods.

As you can tell, using the glycemic index is unlike any diet program you've ever tried. You won't find gimmicks. Instead you'll eat the types of food that let you lose weight and keep it off.

Here's what using the glycemic index for weight loss offers you:

♦ Wholesome and delicious foods that are readily available and highly satisfying. You can be a gourmet cook or a person who prefers to eat prepared foods, and you'll still be able to use the glycemic index.

♦ Reduced food cravings. Of course, you may still want that special piece of chocolate or slice of bread, and you can eat it occasionally without guilt.

♦ Help maintaining balanced energy levels throughout the day.

♦ Help reducing stress by lowering *cortisol levels*. The kinds of food you eat actually help reduce stress. High cortisol levels lead to weight gain, so keeping your stress levels low is a big benefit.

♦ Some treat foods. You can factor in your favorite treats to your daily food intake and enjoy eating them while still losing weight.

Glyco Lingo

Cortisol levels are high when a person's short or long-term stress is high. Elevated cortisol levels often lead to such chronic conditions as weight gain, diabetes, heart disease, cancer, and high blood pressure.

♦ The kinds of food you eat when you lose weight are the same foods you'll eat after you've attained your ideal size. You can stick with low- and moderate-glycemic eating for life.

♦ Improved health. Low-glycemic eating improves health in general and reduces the risk of chronic disease conditions.

Information about eating based on the glycemic index is fast becoming widely available. You'll find information on the Internet and in some popular diet books. We predict that the popularity of the glycemic index is only beginning and will last for a very long time. Your choice of using the glycemic index as a basis for eating and weight loss is a wise and sound decision.

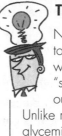

Thin-spiration

No diet should force you to live your life constantly worrying about having "special foods." That's not our definition of special. Unlike many diets, using the glycemic index is lifestyle-friendly. It influences the foods you eat, but it never makes eating seem unpleasant or depressing.

Glycemic Index Basics

Before you can delve into the exquisite and elegant weight loss resources of the glycemic index, you need to know the basics of what it is and what it means.

Here's a simple definition: The *glycemic index* is a scientific measurement of how a person's blood sugar levels change while eating different types of carbohydrate foods. The glycemic index's ranking system is only for carbohydrates and not for proteins or fats.

By itself, the glycemic index isn't an eating program; it's just a method of measuring the impact of carbohydrates on the body. But it is critical for following a healthy eating program. Initially the index was used as a guide for persons with diabetes to help keep their blood sugar levels in the healthy range. Since then, it's been used for weight loss and weight management.

Body of Knowledge

Although the glycemic index is used to measure how carbohydrates affect blood sugar levels and insulin levels, the amount of proteins and fats you eat with carbohydrates can affect blood sugar levels in the body. They're intertwined. High blood sugar levels can ultimately cause weight gain. You'll learn more later in this chapter.

A Brief History

During the 1980s the very low-fat craze took hold, and people were encouraged by health and nutrition experts to eat lots of grains, pastas, and breads whether processed or not. For many individuals the approach backfired. High-carb, especially if it is of the high-glycemic variety, proved to be especially detrimental to persons with diabetes. While eating low fat, they weren't able to maintain stable blood sugar levels because they were eating high-glycemic foods, and, to make matters worse, they gained weight. Persons with diabetes weren't alone. The high-carb, very low-fat approach to eating added many extra inches to the waists of countless individuals. Eating 20 to 30 percent of your diet as fat is considered eating low fat and is recommended in this book. Very low-fat eating is below 20 percent and is not recommended.

Body of Knowledge

Type 2 diabetes is a serious problem in the United States and worldwide. Today, many children and young adults even have Type 2 diabetes. To stay healthy and control their chronic health condition, persons with diabetes need to keep their blood sugar levels within the normal range of 70 to 120 and stable. They can do this through diet, exercise, oral medications, and sometimes by using an insulin-based medication. Their pancreas produces insulin, but the body can't use it. Type 1 diabetes often starts in childhood and is caused when the pancreas is damaged or can't produce adequate amounts of insulin.

That's when Thomas M. S. Wolever, M.D., Ph.D., a professor in the Department of Nutritional Sciences at the University of Toronto in Canada, began conducting research on the effect of carbohydrates on a person's blood sugar levels. His studies were focused on people with Type 2 diabetes. This is often known as adult-onset diabetes.

In his research, Dr. Wolever found that some carbohydrates increased blood sugar levels and, simultaneously, insulin levels, yet some carbohydrates didn't have the same effect. He wanted to discover which foods helped keep blood sugar levels more stable. His explorations led him to design a method for measuring the blood sugar–raising effect of different carbohydrates. The glycemic index was born.

Soon Jennie Brand-Miller, Ph.D., a professor at the University of Sydney in Australia, joined in the research. She has written a whole series of books in the Glucose Revolution series.

Their research and publications have helped thousands and thousands of people control their diabetes through diet. But the value of their research has extended far beyond that to people who want to lose weight and others who want increased good health.

The glycemic index as a basis of dietary and nutritional requirements is widely accepted among health professionals and dietitians in Canada and Australia. Although the United States medical community has been slow to formally recognize the glycemic index, many health-care practitioners now recommend it to their patients. It's also mentioned and recommended in many of the most popular diet books including *SugarBusters!*, *The Zone*, *The South Beach Diet*, and *The New Atkins Diet Revolution*.

Experimental Findings

The glycemic index has excellent credibility and scientific validity because it's been experimentally tested on people—lots of people. Here's a brief overview of how the testing was done and how the glycemic index scale was set up.

Researchers used pure glucose as a baseline standard for the effect that carbohydrates have on blood sugar. First, the blood sugar levels of the research volunteers were tested. Then the volunteers were given glucose to drink. Yes, pure glucose. Although not something found in the average kitchen pantry, glucose is a thick and sweet, though palatable, liquid. About a half-hour later, blood sugar levels were retested. The difference in blood sugar levels told the researchers the amount of glucose needed to cause a rise in blood sugar. Not surprisingly, it was a lot.

The researchers then arbitrarily set the glycemic index of glucose to 100. This established a reference to analyze other foods. The researchers started testing other carbohydrates on their volunteers. They discovered wildly different effects. The glycemic index of carbohydrates tested ranged widely, from almost 0 to 165.

By using the glycemic index as a reference when you eat, you actually know how a food will affect your weight and health. With many food theories, such as food combining or vegetarian eating, personal testimonials are often the only evidence. And, these are often based on a person's internal belief systems and perhaps a desire to prove a point (or not). With actual testing, well, let's put it this way—it would have been difficult and most likely impossible for a volunteer to fool the blood sugar test.

Body of Knowledge

Carbs of all sorts have been given "scores" on the glycemic index. Some lettuces are very low on the glycemic index and are given a glycemic index rank of 0. The highest ranking carb is a tofu frozen dessert at 115.

Research Methods

Early testing of the glycemic effect was a bit inconsistent, but methods for determining the glycemic index of a food have become standardized. Consequently, some early glycemic index lists are now out-of-date and have been revised.

An early test indicated that carrots were high-glycemic. When you think about this, it doesn't make sense. All vegetables are low-glycemic, so why would carrots be high? Recent standardized testing puts cooked carrots at 47 and raw carrot juice at 43. Both are low-glycemic and this makes more sense.

Here's how the testing is now done. Foods are tested on groups of eight to ten people. They consume a standard serving of a carbohydrate in 10 to 15 minutes. A blood sample is taken before the meal and every 15 minutes after for one hour. Then one is taken every 30 minutes for the next hour. Results are inputted into a computer for analysis.

At another time, the volunteers do the same test as above, but this time with pure glucose, because pure glucose provides the baseline for the glycemic index. Pure glucose is 100. The computer analyzes the results, giving a value for the food tested based on the value compared to 100.

The glycemic index of any carbohydrate is an average of the effect on the individuals tested. The real change in blood sugar levels of a specific carbohydrate varies by person, but the variations follow the pattern established by the index. In other words, it's reliable.

Classifications of Carbohydrates

As you know from previous dieting experiences, carbohydrates are present in a wide variety of foods. The glycemic index has been used to develop a very comprehensive list that ranks virtually all the available edible carbohydrates. The sources of carbohydrates are the following:

♦ Starches. This includes all foods made from starches, such as bread, flour, oatmeal, breakfast cereals, white potatoes, rice, tortillas, cookies, pasta, pizza, donuts, and muffins. Starches can be refined or unrefined. In addition, starches include vegetables such as white and sweet potatoes, yams, corn, and winter squash.

♦ Sugars. Including naturally occurring honey and molasses, plus table sugar, fruit sugar (called fructose), and milk sugars (called lactose and galactose). Also included in this category are sodas, shakes, electrolyte-replenishment drinks, lattes, cappuccinos, and other beverages that contain calories. Candy and candy bars are in the sugar category.

◆ Fruits. This category includes all fruit, from apples and pears to pineapple, watermelon, and pomegranates, and fruit juices.

◆ Vegetables. This category contains all vegetables, from lettuces and radishes to summer squash and carrots.

◆ Nuts and seeds. These are combination foods. They contain mostly fat, but also some carbohydrates and protein. Nuts and seeds that don't contain any net carbohydrates, such as pecans and macadamia nuts, aren't tested, because their GI is zero. Two exceptions are cashews and peanuts, as they do contain enough carbohydrates to be tested. Both are low-glycemic.

◆ Dairy products. This category includes mostly milk, yogurt, cream, and ice milk. Some dairy products also contain fat, and some a fair amount of animal protein.

◆ Legumes. Lentils, soy, peanuts, and pinto beans are carbohydrates. Peanuts are considered to be a fat in diabetic exchange booklets, but they also contain carbohydrates, and their glycemic index is low at 14.

Many foods contain combinations of the previous categories and the glycemic index of many processed foods and combination foods are available. See Appendix B for information on where to find glycemic index values for most foods.

High, Medium, and Low

After researchers created a baseline by assigning glucose a value of 100, they assigned a score to all the other carbohydrates, either higher or lower than 100. Carbohydrates with a glycemic index of 55 or lower are considered low-glycemic; those from 56 to 69 are medium-glycemic; those 70 or higher are high-glycemic. You'll find a comprehensive listing of the glycemic index of foods in Appendix B, but here are some general guidelines:

◆ Some cookies have high-glycemic values, and some have mid-level values. Ice cream typically falls in the middle, although some are low. The glycemic index values for these kinds of products vary. They vary based on the amount and type of ingredients. That's why it's best to check with a glycemic index list before you eat.

Thin-spiration

Even though watermelon is high glycemic, it consists of more water and air than carbs. It's a healthy food and contains vitamins, minerals, and antioxidants, so go ahead and enjoy eating watermelon, but eat in moderation, meaning eat no more than one cup per day.

Wrong Weigh

Some foods, such as honey and rice, vary in their glycemic index value. Some varieties of rice are high, some are low, and some are medium. The same is true for honey. The tested values differ based on where the foods were produced, what varieties were tested, and other factors we don't yet understand.

◆ High-glycemic foods include breads, rice crackers, some cookies and cakes, most muffins, and most foods made with enriched white flour. The more easily digestible the starches and sugars in a food, the higher it is on the glycemic index. Refined grain products are usually high as well as most breakfast cereals, white potatoes, and modified food starch. The only fruit that's high glycemic is watermelon and its value is 72.

◆ Medium-glycemic foods include stone-ground breads that don't contain white flour, whole-grain cereals, some cakes and cookies, corn taco shells, table sugar, and energy bars. Some tropical fruits, such as papaya and pineapple, are medium-glycemic.

◆ Low-glycemic foods include all vegetables, most fruits, some whole-grain products such as steel-cut oats and whole barley, and al dente pasta. Legumes, such as lentils and pinto beans, are low-glycemic. Dark chocolate is, too, with a glycemic index of 48. Nuts and seeds are low or 0, and most dairy products, provided they don't have added sugar, are also low.

In your weight-loss program based on the glycemic index, you'll eat carbohydrates that are high-, medium-, and low-glycemic, but you'll mostly eat the ones that are low.

The Least You Need to Know

◆ The glycemic index was developed in the 1980s as a way to quantify how carbohydrates affect blood sugar levels.

◆ Eating in alignment with the glycemic index promotes improved health, lower blood sugar levels, and weight loss.

◆ The glycemic index is receiving recognition worldwide, but has been slower to catch on in the United States. That is now changing rapidly.

◆ Carbohydrates are broadly categorized by the glycemic index as high-, medium-, or low-glycemic.

The Glycemic Index and Insulin Levels

In This Chapter

- ◆ Benefiting from carbohydrates
- ◆ Learning the dynamics of carbohydrates and insulin
- ◆ Pairing stress with insulin
- ◆ Having high insulin levels can cause health conditions

By now you know that carbohydrates are a fascinating category of food. You've been told for years to eat your vegetables, which are carbohydrates and low-glycemic. You're also probably aware that most comfort and treat foods are usually high-glycemic carbohydrates that should be eaten sparingly, if at all. And you know how hard it can be to pass up those enticing high-glycemic donuts, birthday cakes, and pretzels that seem to show up at all parties and events.

In this chapter, you learn more about how carbohydrate consumption relates to health. By understanding the health risks associated with high-carbohydrate and high-glycemic intake, you will strengthen your resolve to attain your ideal size and maintain it.

Health-Giving Carbohydrates

Every day, newspapers, the Internet, and television applaud the health benefits of fruits and vegetables. You're advised to eat 5 to 10 servings a day. That seems like a lot but actually is less than you might think. A serving for nonstarchy vegetables, such as broccoli, is considered to be one cup uncooked or ¹/₂ cup cooked. A serving for fruit is generally ¹/₂ cup or four ounces.

Glyco Lingo

Phytonutrients are the nutrients found in plants and plant products, such as vegetables, fruits, nuts, and seeds. Phytonutrients include vitamins, minerals, antioxidants, and glyconutrients.

There are good reasons the experts recommend you eat carbohydrates. Vegetables and fruits are valuable to you and important for your health. In addition to dietary fiber, plant foods, including nuts and seeds, provide important *phytonutrients*.

Many vegetables have very few grams of carbohydrates in a serving and they're low-glycemic. Most fruits are low-glycemic, some are medium-glycemic, and only watermelon is high-glycemic.

In the information that follows you'll learn about the nutritional goodness found in vegetables and fruits.

Wrong Weigh

When eating your daily 5 to 10 servings of vegetables and fruits, be sure to keep your eating within the boundary of your allotted glycemic load for the day. You'll learn more about the glycemic load in Chapter 5. But for now, know that eating five servings of fruit at one sitting won't work. Neither will eating five servings of starchy vegetables, such as legumes, winter squash, sweet potatoes, corn, and lima beans all at once.

Fiber

You should consume about 25 to 50 grams of dietary fiber every day. Fiber increases the transit time of food in the digestive system, keeps your bowel movements regular, and helps remove toxins from your body quickly. Fiber also gives you a sense of satiation when you eat that helps prevent overeating. But wait, there's even more good news about fiber! Eating foods high in fiber can reduce the effective glycemic index of your meal. And the more fiber in the food, the lower the glycemic index. That's one of the reasons whole-grain breads are lower than white bread in the glycemic index.

> **Wrong Weigh** _____
>
> Although some people may try to receive the full nutritional value of vegetables and fruits by taking dietary supplements, research indicates that it's best to actually consume these gifts from the garden rather than bypass their innate goodness by simply swallowing pills. Think of vitamin/mineral/antioxidant supplements as nutritional insurance. You can certainly take them but, as your mom always said, "Eat your vegetables!"

Try this little imaginary experiment. Picture yourself hungry and gobbling down a half dozen glazed donuts in just a couple of minutes, but then not feeling "satisfied" 20 minutes later. Plausible, right? Now imagine trying to eat an amount of high-fiber celery that contains a comparable total carbohydrate count. Guess how much that would be? You would need to eat more than 90 cups of diced celery to equal the total carb count of 6 donuts! You would feel full after about 20 minutes of eating celery and still have about three days worth of chewing celery to go! The lesson: High-fiber carbs with low-carb counts fit into a healthy diet.

So eat foods high in fiber. And only carbohydrates contain fiber. Neither fats nor animal proteins, such as meat, seafood, dairy, eggs, and cheese, contain fiber. You could take a fiber supplement, but fiber within the foods you eat seems to do more to lower the glycemic index. You get the extra benefit of the nutrients consumed. Taking a fiber supplement at the same time that you eat meals, take medications, or take supplements can block absorption of some nutrients and medications.

Vitamins and Minerals

Consider vegetables and fruits to be your vitamin and mineral warehouse. The water-soluble vitamins, such as vitamin C and the B vitamins, need to be replenished daily because they are either used or flushed from the body continuously. Your body doesn't store these vitamins. This is why you need to eat vegetables and fruits daily. B vitamins are also present in meat and other animal protein, so you can also get them when you eat your moderate serving of animal proteins.

Your body needs a plethora of minerals. The primary ones are calcium, phosphorus, and

> **Body of Knowledge**
>
> Not all vitamins are water-soluble. Vitamins A and E are not. They're stored in fat in the body. These vitamins are also present in vegetables, meats, dairy, fish, and eggs.

Glyco Lingo

Major minerals are those that we require our bodies to ingest in at least an amount of 100 mg (1/50 of a teaspoon). Any other mineral is considered to be a **trace mineral** because the body only needs very small amounts of it.

Wrong Weigh

Antioxidant supplements sometimes work, but occasionally they can actually create more free-radical damage. If you choose to take antioxidant supplements, first research the pros and cons of taking each antioxidant as a supplement. Be careful not to take more than the maximum amount recommended; too high an amount can be harmful.

Glyco Lingo

Glyconutrients are sugars that naturally occur in plants. Some, such as lactose (a milk sugar) and fructose (in fruit) taste sweet. Others include the short chain frutooligosaccharides from foods such as onions and stachyose found in legumes. These are not as sweet. All are needed by the body for important metabolic processes.

magnesium. Your body also needs *trace minerals* such as zinc, iron, chromium, copper, vanadium, manganese, potassium, molybdenum, lithium, cadmium, and boron. (Added all together, it sounds like just about every element from the periodic chart in high school chemistry!) You can find them in the vegetables you eat, as well as from animal protein. You may not need more than tiny amounts of some of the trace elements, but without them, your body's metabolic processes won't work as well.

Antioxidants

Discoveries of new antioxidants occur almost weekly. Once virtually unknown, antioxidants are now front-page news. They protect our bodies from the ravages of free radicals. These free radicals can wreak havoc on bodily functions and immune systems. Damage from free radicals has been implicated in cancer, mood disorders, and degenerative diseases.

Vegetables and fruits are loaded with healthful antioxidants, such as alpha-lipoic acid, glutathione, bioflavinoids, lycopene, and many more. You will also find antioxidants in many popular spices and herbs, which are also carbohydrates. Several supplements contain antioxidants, but you need to use them cautiously and not overconsume them.

Glyconutritionals

Scientists are discovering a whole new branch of carbohydrate chemistry involving *glyconutrients*. They have identified eight special *saccharides* that strengthen the immune system, improve certain health conditions such as autoimmune disorders, help control the stress response, and reduce allergic reactions.

Glyconutrients are present in fruits and vegetables but are not present in any significant amounts in processed high-glycemic carbohydrates. One glyconutrient you may have heard of is beta-1, 3-glucan, which is useful for treating many bacterial, viral, and fungal diseases, as well as killing tumor cells and increasing bone-marrow production.

Because glyconutrients exhibit such powerful immune-system modulation ability, many pharmaceutical companies are developing medications using glyconutrients. You can also purchase nutritional supplements containing these important nutrients. You may want to use supplements, but you already get the benefits of glyconutrients when you eat a wide variety of vegetables and fruits.

Stay tuned as more information on the wonderful health-giving aspects of glyconutrients becomes available. They give you even more reasons to eat your carbohydrates.

Glyco Lingo

Saccharides is the scientific term for sugars. The term includes all sugars, including the sugars we normally eat, such as sucrose, fructose, and lactose (the sugar in milk). Saccharides also include other lesser-known sugars present in foods that don't raise blood sugar levels, which are considered non-nutritive because they don't contain calories.

A Gourmet Palate

Another very important advantage of eating your vegetables and fruits is that they make eating more interesting. A daily diet of animal protein and fat would become boring in less than a day. But with vegetables and fruits, food becomes palatable, colorful, and tasty.

Just imagine food without spices, without salsa, without herbs, without pesto. Such a dull life. Imagine no recipes, no garnishes, no pickles, and no ethnic cuisine. No one would even want to eat, except to sustain life.

Carbohydrates save us from palate boredom. The varied fragrances whet our appetites and make mealtimes much more pleasurable. Hurrah for this aspect of carbs!

The Regulatory Hormone, Insulin

Think of insulin as a highly beneficial hormone. It literally keeps you alive. But again, too much of a good thing—in this case, insulin—is damaging. You want to have enough insulin in your body to keep you thin and healthy and not so much that you fall prey to its dire health consequences.

Insulin is the hormone that regulates blood sugar levels. It delivers energy in the form of both sugar and fat to your body's cells. The pancreas gland excretes insulin when you eat food. Carbohydrates cause the biggest impact with insulin secretion, and the higher the glycemic index of the carbohydrate, and the more you eat of it, the more insulin the pancreas pumps out. When you eat low-glycemic carbohydrates, on the other hand, the pancreas secrete less insulin. Too much insulin in your bloodstream becomes a health problem. This condition is called hyperinsulinism. This happens when …

Glyco Lingo

Glycemic load is a calculation of the amount of a carbohydrate food factored by the glycemic index of the food. This number gives you a good sense of how what you eat will affect your blood sugar levels and insulin levels.

Glyco Lingo

Insulin resistant is a medical and biological term that means the body's cells do not respond properly to insulin. They don't uptake glucose and fat efficiently. When this happens, a person has too much insulin in the blood stream. This leads to weight gain, metabolic syndrome, and often Type 2 diabetes.

♦ You eat too many high-glycemic carbohydrates. Insulin levels surge beyond your body's need for cellular energy. In the case of high-glycemic carbs, it doesn't take much to trigger too much insulin production. On the other hand, if you eat too many low-glycemic carbs you can also trigger too much insulin secretion. You'll learn how to balance your carb intake with the glycemic index of food in Chapter 5.

♦ You eat too high a *glycemic load* for a long period of time, as in months and years. Your body's cells become resistant to the insulin, or *insulin resistant*, thus requiring the pancreas to produce more and more insulin to deliver sugar and fat to your cells for energy.

♦ Your stress levels are high. The stress hormone cortisol causes an increase in insulin.

♦ If you are a person with Type 2 diabetes or with impaired glucose tolerance, also known as borderline diabetes, your body may no longer be able to uptake blood sugar into the cells. The body usually produces enough insulin, but your body cannot use the insulin efficiently. Consequently, your blood sugar levels stay too high.

◆ You eat too much food. Continually overeating increases your insulin levels even if you're not overeating only carbohydrates. You can still overproduce insulin by overeating protein or fat.

◆ Fasting, not eating or skipping meals, can cause insulin resistance.

When you have elevated levels of insulin in your body, the excess insulin can cause low blood sugar. This can make you lightheaded, jittery, and anxious and is anything but desirable.

Weight Gain

Insulin is the hormone that causes the body to store fat. When blood sugar levels surge, insulin converts the excess sugar into fat in the form of triglycerides. Some of these triglycerides are moved into storage in your fat cells. And of course, you gain weight. Unfortunately, stored fat tends to stick around for a while.

By keeping your insulin levels low and avoiding hyperinsulinism, your body stops storing excess energy as fat. Instead your body uses your stored fat as fuel, and you lose weight. This occurs most efficiently on a low–glycemic index weight-loss program. Even after you lose weight and reach your ideal size, you should avoid overstimulation of insulin production. Your maintenance phase needs to focus on keeping your insulin levels low to avoid regaining weight.

Type 2 Diabetes

Some people with Type 2 diabetes also have elevated levels of insulin. Unfortunately, their diabetes prevents their bodies from efficiently delivering energy-giving sugars and fats to their cells. Their blood sugar levels remain elevated. This leads to damaged blood vessels, which may cause eye disease, heart disease, early dementia, nerve damage to the limbs and internal organs, and kidney disease. In addition, diabetics often continue to gain weight, leading to obesity, which has its own set of health risks.

It's easy to see why a glycemic index weight-loss program is almost always recommended for individuals with Type 2 diabetes. It helps lower blood sugar and insulin levels so they can manage their condition and become healthier.

At your annual physical examination, ask your doctor to test for elevated blood sugar levels. The sooner a person discovers he or she is at risk for Type 2 diabetes, the easier it is to control the condition and avoid its debilitating consequences.

High LDL Cholesterol

In addition to increasing blood sugar, excess levels of insulin increase triglycerides. Also, as a person gains weight, there's normally an increase in the LDL count. LDL is the so-called bad cholesterol. A high LDL count indicates a higher risk of heart attacks than a low LDL.

For many years health professionals believed that a diet high in saturated fats caused high cholesterol and heart disease. Now we know that the cause and effect is more complex. Eating lots of high-glycemic carbohydrates can also cause elevated lipid levels and heart disease. Eating smaller amounts of carbohydrates and eating low-glycemic carbohydrates appears to boost the good cholesterol (HDL).

In addition, eating too much saturated fat and *trans-fatty acids*, or partially hydrogenated vegetable oils, also causes clogged arteries and heart disease.

Glyco Lingo

Trans-fatty acids are man-made by converting unsaturated vegetable oils into partially hydrogenated vegetable oils through heating. Partially hydrogenated fats are solids at room temperature and are more chemically stable, meaning that they have a longer shelf life than an unsaturated vegetable oil. Trans-fatty acids have been shown to directly cause clogged arteries and heart disease. They are found in many commercially available baked goods and other processed foods. The FDA is requiring that all food labels list the amount of trans-fats per serving.

For the best results, limit the saturated fat in your diet, avoid all partially hydrogenated vegetable oils and trans-fats, eat meals that contain low-glycemic carbohydrates, keep your glycemic load within your goals, and avoid or drink sparingly all alcoholic beverages.

Body of Knowledge

Eating too many carbohydrates, eating too many high-glycemic carbohydrates, and drinking too much alcohol will also increase your triglyceride level. To keep triglyceride levels low, a woman should not drink more than one 3-ounce serving of wine or the equivalent in one day. Men should have no more than two 3-ounce servings of wine or the equivalent. However, because drinking alcohol beverages can also affect your ability to lose weight, you may want to avoid alcohol altogether.

Thick Artery Walls

Elevated insulin levels cause the artery walls to grow thicker, which in effect narrows the diameter of the passageway. This makes it more likely that cholesterol will adhere inside the walls and lead to blocked arteries and heart disease.

As the passageways of the arteries get narrower, blood pressure increases. Alas, insulin also has other ways of increasing a person's blood pressure.

Kidney Function

When insulin levels are elevated, insulin sends signals to the kidneys to hold on to salt. The kidneys comply and then do even more because the kidneys need to maintain a proper saline balance in the body. To do that, the kidneys retain enough water to balance out the increased salt reserves.

The result is that you gain water weight, which increases your blood pressure. Although water weight isn't the same as an increase in body fat, it still adds pounds and tightens the fit on your clothes.

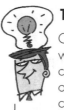

Thin-spiration

On a glycemic-savvy weight-loss program, you could lose several pounds of water weight in the first couple of weeks. This is good because it can help lower high blood pressure. Don't be concerned; you'll also be losing fat, and your fat loss will continue as your water weight stabilizes.

Inflammation

Inflammation is another health-related consequence of elevated insulin levels. Many medical experts believe inflammation is a major cause of disease. These diseases may include cancer, Alzheimer's, acne, skin rashes, and autoimmune diseases such as allergies, asthma, fibromyalgia, multiple sclerosis, and arthritis. Even aging is thought to be a function of inflammation. (If this proves true, then maybe eating based on the glycemic index will become a veritable Fountain of Youth!)

Research indicates that lowering insulin levels can help prevent inflammation and the resultant disease conditions. The best way to do that is to eat based on the glycemic index.

Magnesium Deficiency

Magnesium is a necessary mineral used by the body to relax muscles, including the muscles of the arteries. It also eases muscle cramps. When insulin levels are elevated because of insulin resistance, however, the body stores less magnesium. Less magnesium in the body means that the blood vessels are more likely to be constricted, which leads to high blood pressure.

It's a vicious cycle. When your body lacks adequate amounts of magnesium, you have less energy, which can lead to overeating and even binge eating. Eating foods that are low-glycemic will enhance your intake of magnesium. Whole, unprocessed grains and low-glycemic foods are often high in many nutrients, including magnesium.

Polycystic Ovary Syndrome

When a woman's ovaries are exposed to too much insulin, polycystic ovary syndrome (PCOS) can occur. This leads to the ovaries producing too much of the hormones testosterone and androstene. In the United States, 1 in 10 obese women have PCOS. It leads to hair loss, acne, and infertility. It also puts women at high risk for heart disease and Type 2 diabetes.

The bottom line is that keeping your insulin levels in a normal range not only helps you lose weight and enjoy living at your ideal size, it definitely helps you stay healthy.

Stress and Insulin Levels

Adrenaline and cortisol are often referred to as the "stress hormones." That's because your body produces these hormones under stress. Unfortunately, cortisol has been shown to cause weight gain when our bodies produce too much of it. Insulin and the stress hormones are, in effect, team players. They need each other. When insulin levels are elevated, so are the levels of adrenaline and cortisol. The reverse is also true. When your stress levels are high, your insulin levels are elevated.

What this means is that it's best if you can keep your stress levels low. Elevated stress levels contribute to health concerns.

- Cortisol overload causes weight gain in your midsection—the area around your waist.

- Cortisol overload breaks down muscle, thus causing your basal metabolic rate to slow down.

♦ Because cortisol overload reduces the number of muscle cells, a person has fewer cells to uptake blood sugar, so more sugar gets stored as fat, increasing body fat levels.

♦ Cortisol uses up brain chemicals, also known as neurotransmitters. When the brain neurotransmitter serotonin is depleted, a person can have difficulty sleeping and can experience depression and anxiety. The feelings of depression and anxiety can lead to activities that further increase stress, such as smoking, drinking caffeine, using alcoholic beverages, and eating high-glycemic foods for comfort.

High stress always makes weight loss more difficult. If your stress levels are high, you may not be able to lose weight as quickly as you want, even on a glycemic-savvy weight-loss program. When you reduce your stress, you'll lose more quickly. In Chapter 23, you learn how to reduce stress and relax more so that you can keep your insulin levels low.

The Least You Need to Know

♦ Carbohydrates benefit your health by providing fiber, vitamins, minerals, anti-oxidants, and glyconutrients.

♦ Elevated insulin levels cause weight gain and promote chronic health conditions and diseases.

♦ A weight-loss program that is based on low-glycemic eating helps you lose weight and keep your insulin levels in a healthy range.

♦ High insulin levels increase the stress hormone cortisol, which can also lead to weight gain.

Glycemic Index Weight-Loss Benefits

In This Chapter

- ◆ Experiencing higher energy levels
- ◆ Reducing hunger and cravings
- ◆ Managing your moods
- ◆ Having extra feel-good body perks
- ◆ Eating comfortably with others

Just the mention of the word *dieting* can bring back dreadful memories of past experiences and failures. If you dieted by reducing your caloric intake, you might have felt like you were starving. You probably tried valiantly to wrestle with and overcome your incredibly intense food cravings. You might also remember feeling bloated and constipated.

Stepping on scales occasionally gave you joyful highs but it more likely provoked self-doubt, lowered your self-esteem, and increased your anxiety. You, and others you loved, endured your dramatic and uncontrollable mood swings as your blood sugar levels plummeted midmorning and late afternoon. Of course, you were delighted when your clothes became looser and you could fit into a smaller pair of jeans—at least, temporarily—but you may have noticed that your appearance took on an unhealthy pallor.

The good news is that those dieting days are in your past. The "good old days" of deprivation dieting, when experts thought depriving yourself of food was the only way to lose weight, are over. With a glycemic index weight-loss program, you won't feel as if you're starving or suffering emotionally. In fact, you can lose weight while realizing terrific lifestyle and health benefits. In this chapter, you'll learn all about them.

Personal Gains

Glycemic index weight loss is exciting because it helps you feel good. Doesn't that just seem right? When you're doing good things for your body, such as losing weight, shouldn't you feel good throughout the entire process? Absolutely. Ideally, you should feel at least as good, if not better, than you feel when you aren't on a weight-loss program at all. That's what glycemic index weight loss has to offer!

With glycemic index weight loss, you can experience personal gains in day-to-day energy levels and drop pounds at the same time. You'll not only see the difference in how your clothes fit, you'll also notice a positive difference in the appearance of your skin, hair, and nails. You'll even find that your moods are brighter and more stable. And, as an added bonus, your stress levels are likely to be reduced.

How is all this possible? Glycemic-savvy eating actually changes the way your body works.

Energy Levels

You want to have energy to burn, and you can. Your body already has abundant energy stored as fat. Glycemic index weight loss lets you access that stored fat and burn it for fuel. On many other kinds of diets, your body burns muscle for energy. When you limit carbohydrate intake, however, your body uses up stored fat with less muscle loss.

All your excess weight is, in essence, stored energy, and with a glycemic index eating plan, you finally get to live off of your body fat and use it up. You can't just stop eating and live entirely on stored fat. But by eating correctly while losing weight, you may finally "burn off" body fat you already have stored *and* keep your energy levels high for months.

Some of the specific benefits of increased energy levels are as follows:

♦ Say good-bye to late-afternoon energy slumps. Those have been caused by blood sugar and insulin level swings. Your blood sugar levels will become more stable throughout the day.

♦ You'll notice an increase in mental alertness. You'll have a steady supply of energy going to your brain from the energy supplied by fat burning, whereas energy from uneven blood sugar levels can contribute to *brain fog*.

> **Glyco Lingo**
>
> **Brain fog** is an unscientific term that describes the condition in which a person has difficulty thinking or behaving coherently. At those times a person could misplace keys—or children—and forget to do everyday chores. The person feels as if his IQ has dropped. This is often caused by low blood sugar levels, but it can also be caused by other more serious health conditions.

♦ Insulin resistance you have abates, so your body's cells can uptake more energy. If you've had periods of fatigue in the past caused by insulin resistance, expect them to diminish.

When you have more energy, you naturally participate in more activities. This contributes to further weight loss and starts a very positive upward spiral for weight loss and lifestyle success.

Eating Patterns

If you've been on a restricted-calorie diet before, you know how hard it is to avoid overeating when you feel hungry all the time. Throw in the sudden and unexpected food cravings that can make a mess of your best intentions, and it's easy to see why staying on a restricted-calorie diet is agonizingly difficult and certainly not fun. On a glycemic index weight-loss program, however, it is easier to avoid both overeating and the horrendous, and at times irresistible, food cravings. That kind of hunger is induced by the restrictive nature of those diets.

Natural hunger—the kind you experience when your body actually needs food—is good because it signals that it's time to eat. But your natural hunger feelings can easily get confused with false hunger. False hunger comes when you feel compelled to eat more food than your body requires.

False hunger is often the result of swings in insulin levels. When you eat a high-carbohydrate meal or snack, your blood sugar is elevated and you feel satiated. Soon after that, however, your insulin levels increase quickly and lower your blood sugar levels. You feel hungry again. If you respond to this feeling by eating yet more high-glycemic, high-carb foods, you end up in an unsatisfying and fattening cycle. By eating mostly low-glycemic carbohydrates, you eliminate false hunger.

Food cravings are often a result of the same high-carb insulin-hunger cycle. You crave high-carb foods because they quickly increase your blood sugar levels and make you comfortable. Yes, it's usually carbs we crave. Very few of us—if anyone—who's caught up in an insulin-hunger cycle craves a fish fillet or a plain tossed salad. Instead, our cravings range from donuts and cookies to candy and bagels—foods that will keep the insulin-hunger cycle going strong. By avoiding the high-carb foods altogether, you avoid cravings and the insulin-hunger cycle.

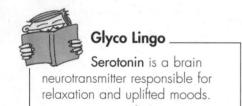

Glyco Lingo

Serotonin is a brain neurotransmitter responsible for relaxation and uplifted moods.

Food cravings are also caused by stress. When times get tough and schedules become hectic, levels of the stress hormone cortisol rise. That's when many of us seek comfort foods such as mashed potatoes, rice pudding, and oatmeal cookies. These are among the foods that seem to lift our moods and soothe our stress, at least temporarily. But why?

These high-carbohydrate foods increase levels of the brain neurotransmitter *serotonin*. Serotonin soothes the brain and makes us feel relaxed. But—you guessed it—there's a downside. These foods make us fat, only work temporarily, and can ultimately increase anxiety and depression.

Here's how. These foods put us back on the insulin-hunger cycle in which our blood sugar is lifted and then crashes as more insulin is delivered to the bloodstream. Insulin and cortisol tend to always stay balanced in the body; so when people are stressed, their insulin level and cortisol level increase, which causes their body to store fat more readily. Ultimately, they gain weight. As insulin increases, so does cortisol. Cortisol uses up serotonin, which results in yet more feelings of anxiety, stress, and depression.

You learn more about how to manage your stress without eating high-glycemic, high-carb foods in Chapter 23. But for now, know that you have plenty of excellent alternatives, ranging from meditation to exercise, and even sleep will restore serotonin levels.

Mood Management

Eating high-glycemic food creates mood disorders. Your body reacts to these foods by increasing insulin levels, which then increases the level of stress hormones.

With elevated levels of adrenaline and corti-sol, a person easily experiences anxiety, panic attacks, and depression. If stress hormones stay high over a long period of time, a person can end up medically diagnosed with a mood disorder.

As you control insulin levels with a glycemic index weight-loss program, you should feel better and have fewer down or anxious moments. This is a great win-win situation for someone trying to lose weight because just being on a weight-loss program often adds stress. So expect to feel good and feel in control of your moods, which makes for great weight-loss success.

> **Thin-spiration**
>
> If you are suffering from serious mood disorders, such as depression, anxi-ety, or bipolar conditions, ask your health practitioner if avoiding high-glycemic, high-carb foods could improve your situation. Many psychiatrists and psychologists now recommend avoiding most high-glycemic starches and other high-glycemic foods as part of an overall men-tal health regimen.

Body Perks

Glycemic index weight loss offers you some terrific physical body benefits that you'll appreciate throughout your weight-loss program, including your maintenance pro-gram. Because we each have unique body chemistry and needs, the following benefits will vary:

♦ **Better and sounder sleep.** Because your stress levels won't be increased due to increased insulin and cortisol, more serotonin will be available, enabling you to get to sleep easier and to sleep more soundly. However, if your stress levels are already high because of other life situations, you might not fully realize this benefit.

♦ **Flatter tummy.** Yes, it takes plenty of exercise, crunches, and sweat to produce abs of steel. But if insulin and cortisol are raging through your body because of the insulin, high-carb connection, your ab crunching efforts may produce paltry results. As your insulin levels stabilize at a lower level, you can expect to see a marked reduction in tummy flab. You can accelerate this result with an exercise program, as described in Part 6.

◆ **Regularity.** Because you'll be eating 25 grams or more of dietary fiber every day, you'll decrease the transit time of food and waste products through your digestive system. (To help everything along, be sure to drink at least the recommended eight glasses of water every day.)

◆ **Fewer plateaus.** Weight-loss plateaus are the bane of people who are on any weight-loss program. You start losing weight but then plateau or level out, and, no matter how rock-steady you are on your diet, you can't seem to lose the next few pounds. The stall seems unfair and can be so disappointing that a person loses momentum and enthusiasm. We can't promise that you won't experience a weight-loss plateau on a glycemic index weight-loss program, but provided you follow the total program, it will be short-lived and perhaps nonexistent.

◆ **Clearer skin.** Who doesn't want to have better skin? Elevated insulin levels can cause inflammation, and the inflammation shows up in many areas of your body. One of them is your skin. Dermatologists now recommend a low-glycemic eating plan along with supplementation of essential fatty acids to improve the appearance of your skin and make it moist, plump, and radiant. Eating right can reduce wrinkling, acne, breakouts, congestion, and other annoying skin conditions. You learn more about essential fatty acids in Chapter 12.

Glyco Lingo

Insulin sensitivity is a term that indicates the body's cells respond to insulin correctly. This is the opposite of insulin resistance, in which the body's cells don't respond adequately to insulin and therefore don't absorb nutrients, such as blood sugar, efficiently.

◆ **Fewer allergic reactions.** Research shows that people who eat meals based on the glycemic index tend to have fewer allergies or display milder symptoms. This is because lower insulin levels enhance immune system function. Is it possible that you'll have fewer colds? We can't promise you, but it's possible.

◆ **Aging.** An important contributor to longevity is *insulin sensitivity*. Insulin sensitivity means your cells are responding to insulin and correctly uptaking blood sugar for energy. By keeping your insulin levels low, the odds are you'll age better and live longer, too.

Of course, the biggest body perk is that you'll attain your ideal size and be able to stay there for life, simply by continuing to eat mostly low-glycemic foods and meals within the framework of a healthy lifestyle. No matter why you want to lose weight—to look good, for self-esteem, to move on with your life, or to improve your health—you'll have the opportunity to achieve your goals.

Health Benefits

By eating based on the glycemic index, you reduce your risk of …

- Type 2 diabetes.

- Heart disease.

- High cholesterol.

- High blood pressure.

- Autoimmune disease conditions, such as arthritis, allergies, fibromyalgia, and multiple sclerosis.

- Depression and anxiety.

- Alzheimer's and other dementias.

- Some cancers, including breast, colon, rectal, and endometrial cancers.

Research continues on the health benefits of eating based on the glycemic index. In the next few years, expect to read even more about why managing your insulin levels is advantageous to your health.

Feeding the Whole Family

After you learn how to locate, prepare, and eat low-glycemic foods, you'll be delighted with how easy it is. You'll also be amazed at how good the foods taste. You'll learn how to eat in virtually any restaurant and how to prepare meals quickly and simply. We give you plenty of meal ideas later in this book, and you can also use the recipes in *The Complete Idiot's Guide to Low-Carb Meals* and *The Complete Idiot's Guide to Terrific Diabetic Meals* as guides for eating.

With some modifications, your glycemic index weight-loss program can work well for every member of your family. Remember, not only can individuals lose weight by eating mostly low-glycemic foods, they also gain marvelous health benefits. Certainly you want those health benefits for everyone in your family and for all your friends. You can serve low-glycemic foods at parties, take low-glycemic prepared dishes to potluck dinners, and feed your family and friends every day with the same foods you'll be eating on a glycemic index weight-loss plan.

If you have ever been on another type of diet that limited your food choices and your calorie intake, you know that not limiting choices and calories is a terrific benefit to being on a glycemic index weight-loss program. You might have sat at dinner night after night watching your teenage children devour pizzas or burgers while you ate a slice of Melba toast, some dry chicken breast, and a small green salad dressed with lemon juice. Not any longer.

It's much more fun to fit in when you eat with others and not draw attention to yourself and your food needs. Now you won't have to. You'll need to learn a few "tricks" and techniques—which come later in the book—but you don't have to feel like the oddball at any meal.

The Least You Need to Know

- ◆ Your energy levels will be higher and more balanced when you are on a glycemic index weight-loss program.

- ◆ You avoid the intense hunger and food cravings of other types of dieting when eating low-glycemic foods.

- ◆ Glycemic index weight-loss programs help you reduce stress, improve sleep, and minimize dieting plateaus.

- ◆ Your overall health will improve with a glycemic index weight-loss program.

What Makes a Carbohydrate Low-Glycemic

In This Chapter

◆ Learning glycemic index food facts

◆ Comparing good carbs and bad carbs

◆ Identifying digestible carbs

◆ Understanding processed and unprocessed carbohydrates

The world of carbohydrates seems to come with its own vocabulary. You've heard such terms as complex carbohydrates and refined sugars. Plus, you've probably heard that there are "bad carbs" and "good carbs," as if carbs are either angelic or demonic. The terms have become part of our collective weight-loss jargon.

Don't worry. There's no reason why "carb talk" has to be weighty, vague, or confusing. You won't need expert knowledge to know which carbohydrates you should eat and which ones to eat sparingly. We make this simple for you to understand.

But it will be highly useful for you to have a fundamental understanding of carbohydrates. The knowledge will help you make wise food choices in your daily life. In this chapter, you learn about the different categories of carbohydrates, and you learn more about how they relate to the glycemic index.

Some Simple Rules of Thumb

As this chapter explains the differences between carbohydrates, keep in mind the following guidelines. Think of them as "rules of thumb" that you need to modify to your personal weight-loss needs:

- The refined carbohydrates are usually high-glycemic. These include foods made from white flour and refined grains.

- White sugar is medium-glycemic, whereas the glycemic index of honey varies based on origin. Single-flower honeys are usually low-glycemic, but those from a mixture of flowers are usually medium-glycemic but can be high-glycemic on occasion.

- Breads made from finely milled enriched white or whole wheat flours are high-glycemic. Rice cakes are also high-glycemic.

- The slower a complex carb breaks down into its simple sugars in your digestive track, the lower-glycemic it is. Stone-ground wheat bread takes more time to digest in your stomach than white bread, so its glycemic index is lower.

- Dietary fiber slows down starch and sugar absorption in the stomach, and so consequently lowers the glycemic index.

Body of Knowledge

Dietary fiber that's actually part of the food, as in brown rice or stone-ground flour, is usually better for lowering the glycemic index of a food rather than adding fiber, such as oat or wheat bran, to refined, finely milled flour. However, if a large portion, $1/3$ to $1/2$ of the total dry ingredients, is unprocessed wheat bran fiber, then the glycemic index can end up being low. For low-glycemic recipes of breads see *The Complete Idiot's Guide to Terrific Diabetic Meals.*

- Naturally occurring unprocessed carbohydrates, such as vegetables, whole kernel grains, and fruits, are lower-glycemic than processed carbohydrates, such as baked goods and candy.

◆ Nutrient-dense carbohydrates are healthier for you because they contain more important vitamins, minerals, antioxidants, and other micronutrients.

As you eat based on the glycemic index, you'll gain an instinctive knowledge about which foods will trigger a rise in your blood sugar levels and which ones won't. Until then, plan your meals with a glycemic index list close at hand.

Body of Knowledge
It's possible that some low-glycemic or medium-glycemic foods react in your body as if they were high-glycemic. Researchers don't know why this happens, but it does. If you suspect a food works differently for you, by all means, eat it carefully. Bananas may seem high-glycemic to you, but actually, they're listed as low at 52.

Easy or Hard to Digest

The faster your body can digest a carbohydrate, the higher its glycemic index value. There are two major types of digestible polysaccharides or complex carbohydrates: amylose and amylopectin. Both contain many glucose units, but the foods with more amylopectin raise the blood glucose levels much more readily than foods containing more amylose. The branches in amylopectin starch have many surface areas, which make it easier for digestive enzymes to break it down faster.

These easy-to-break-down starches include foods such as most breads, white potatoes, white flour, and snack foods such as pretzels, donuts, and cookies. Most of these foods are also processed or refined carbohydrates, but some natural unprocessed carbohydrates have higher amylopectin levels, including parsnips, russet potatoes, and rutabagas.

Starches that contain more amylose include some whole grains and legumes (lentils, dried peas, and beans) and some of the starchy vegetables such as yams and sweet potatoes. These foods are best for your glycemic index weight-loss program.

Dietary Fiber

Most dietary fiber is not digestible. In other words, you might consume the fiber, but there's a good chance most of it will not be digested such that the nutrients enter your bloodstream. Instead, the fiber is excreted in your stool. There are two major types of fiber: soluble and insoluble. Mostly it is the insoluble fiber that does not get digested, but both types of fiber slow the rate of carbohydrate breakdown into blood glucose. Because of this, it's great for you to eat lots of dietary fiber. Ideally, you should consume 25 grams or more every day.

Don't overdo the fiber. But you'd need to consume a virtually unpalatable amount of fiber supplements, such as psyllium husks, to eat too much fiber—such as 4 or 5 tablespoons a day. With too much fiber, you could actually block the absorption of important vitamins, minerals, amino acids, and more. Overeating fiber can, in essence, make you undernourished. (And undernourished doesn't equate to being thinner.) More than 45 grams of fiber a day is generally too much for most of us.

Refined and Unrefined Carbohydrates

Another distinction that some nutritional counselors make is between refined and unrefined carbohydrates. In glycemic index weight loss, we prefer to classify carbohydrates as low-, medium-, or high-glycemic. However, because you're bound to hear carbohydrates defined as refined and unrefined, this section discusses how the terminology relates to the glycemic index.

Refined carbohydrates are more highly processed than unrefined carbohydrates. Processing includes such activities as cooking, milling, and separating the whole food into parts. Examples of refined carbohydrates are white bread, white rice, most packaged breakfast cereals, donuts, cakes, cookies, bagels, fruit and vegetable juices, fruit drinks, soda, and candy. The list goes on. Refined carbs are usually high-glycemic, but some can be low, as in vegetable juice and some fruit juices.

Unrefined carbohydrates are those kept in their natural state. In general, the unrefined carbohydrates tend to contain more fiber. Examples of unrefined carbohydrates are whole vegetables and fruit, whole grains, dried peas and beans, and nuts and seeds. Some foods are processed more than others. For example, fruit juice is not processed as much as fruit drinks. Usually unrefined carbs are low-glycemic, but not always, so be sure to check the glycemic index listings before you eat them.

Pastas

Even though regular pasta is a highly refined, processed carbohydrate, its glycemic value can be low, medium, or high, depending on how you cook it. If you cook spaghetti for only 5 to 6 minutes, it's low-glycemic. Other types of pasta may need slightly more or less cooking time. If you open a can of prepared spaghetti in sauce, those noodles will have a higher glycemic index because they're mushy.

Cook pasta just until it softens and you'll be eating a healthier meal. The longer pasta is cooked the more available the starch in the pasta is for quick digestion—exactly what you don't want.

The Good and the Bad

Carbohydrates aren't good or bad; the difference is in how you eat them and how much of them you eat. This is one of the reasons why glycemic index weight loss works so well. You don't need to give up your favorite treat food, whether it's white bread, bagels, or candy bars. But you do need to eat them in such a way that you don't cause a quick rise in your blood sugar levels, and you do need to watch portion sizes.

The glycemic index gives you a way of managing your blood sugar and insulin levels, thus assuring that you aren't storing fat and also that you continue to lose weight.

One way to do this is to manage your glycemic load by meal and by day. You'll be balancing the low-glycemic foods with some high and some medium, and overall, you can keep your insulin levels low. You'll learn more about the glycemic load in Chapter 5.

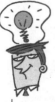

Thin-spiration

Angela loved eating sugar. In fact, she'd never met a sweet treat that she didn't want to eat. Her intense sugar cravings bothered her and she wanted to lose about 30 pounds. She embarked on a glycemic index weight-loss program and decided that it was very easy for her to give up breads and wheat products to eat mostly low-glycemic. But she didn't want to stop all sugary foods. And she didn't need to. In her food plan, she was able to include two ounces of dark chocolate twice a week, and still lose weight.

Now's the time to give up the notion of bad and good carbs and of fattening and non-fattening carbs. Instead, accept all carbs as okay, based on how you eat them.

The Acid Factor

The only way to describe how acidic foods affect the glycemic index is to say it's unexpected. Who would have thought that eating an acidic-tasting food with a carbohydrate would lower the effective glycemic index? Most likely, no one.

Yet, that's exactly what happens. Acidic foods significantly lower the glycemic index of a food or a meal by one-third. The reason lies in how your stomach and digestive system work. Acidic foods slow the emptying of your stomach. The foods slow down your digestion, which slows down how quickly your blood sugar rises.

Yes, this is a wonderful boon to your weight-loss program. You can manage the glycemic effect of your meals by what you eat. Here's a list of foods that are acidic:

- Chutney

- Dill and sweet pickles

- Green olives

- Horseradish

- Lemon juice

- Lime juice

- Marinated vegetables, such as artichokes, mushrooms, carrots, and green beans

- Pickled beets

- Pickled eggs

- Pickled garlic

- Pickled herring

- Pickled legumes

- Pickled peppers, such as jalapeños

- Sauerbraten

- Sauerkraut

- Sourdough bread

- Tangy salsas

- Vinegar

- Vinegar and oil salad dressings

Thin-spiration

If you love croutons on your salads, but don't want to eat the high-glycemic breads, make your own croutons with sourdough bread. Cut the bread into small cubes and lightly sauté in olive oil or butter and spices, such as Italian seasoning. Store them in an airtight bag in the refrigerator. Use just a few—they add great flavor and crunch.

Some of the acidic foods, such as pickled beets, chutney, some of the marinated vegetables, and sweet pickles have added sugar. Consequently, these foods are not recommended in large quantities.

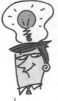

Thin-spiration

In using the glycemic index for weight loss, Sally learned that her body simply couldn't handle white bread. Within minutes of eating it, she would feel bloated and uncomfortable. By the next day, her clothes were tight. This is the case with bread except for sourdough bread. She can eat a small piece of sourdough bread once or twice a week with a complete meal without any side effects or weight gain. The difference is that sourdough bread is acidic.

Use the acidic foods as condiments and side dishes to your meals and snacks. Toss your salads with vinegar and oil salad dressings. You need four teaspoons of vinegar on your salad to reduce the glycemic value of your meal by about 30 percent. Use lemon to flavor your herbal teas and your water at meals. Make guacamole salad with fresh-squeezed lime juice.

Think of a balanced meal as containing animal protein, vegetables, and an acidic food. Your waistline will be glad you did.

Don't Count These Carbs

Some carbohydrates aren't listed in the glycemic index. They simply don't contain enough carbohydrate to affect your blood sugar levels. These are most of the non-starchy vegetables as indicated on the bottom of the new Food Guide Pyramid in this book. On average these vegetables contain about 5 grams of carbohydrates for 1 cup raw or 1/2 cup cooked vegetables. Lettuce varieties, including raw spinach, contain about two grams of carbohydrates per one cup raw lettuce—so for salad greens, use it as a free food.

Body of Knowledge

The spice, cinnamon, has been shown to lower blood glucose levels in persons with diabetes. Here's how to use cinnamon for weight loss. If you add cinnamon as a flavoring to foods, such as sweet potatoes or herbal teas, you could effectively lower the glycemic effect of a meal. But use only small quantities, between 1/4 to 1 teaspoon a day. Don't use larger amounts because one of the flavorings in cinnamon, coumarin, can cause mutations or cancer if eaten in large amounts. The toxic materials in cinnamon are insoluble, so if you want to consume more than what's indicated here, boil the cinnamon in water and pour off the soluble part for use and then discard the solid part.

Here's the list of foods you can eat freely without concern to glycemic index:

- Alfalfa sprouts
- Artichokes
- Asparagus
- Bamboo shoots
- Broccoli
- Cabbage
- Carrots, raw
- Cauliflower
- Celery
- Celery root
- Chard, Swiss
- Collards
- Cucumber
- Eggplant
- Endive
- Fennel
- Green beans
- Hearts of palm
- Jicama
- Kale
- Lettuce
- Mushrooms
- Mustard greens
- Okra
- Onions
- Parsley
- Pea pods
- Peppers
- Radicchio
- Radishes
- Sauerkraut
- Scallions
- Spinach
- Squash, summer
- Squash, zucchini
- Tomatillos
- Tomatoes
- Turnip greens
- Turnips
- Water chestnuts
- Watercress

Some other foods not classified as nonstarchy veggies, but also very low in carbohydrates and with a "0" glycemic index, include the following:

- Avocados—Serving size for avocados are $1/4$ small. Even though it is a 0 glycemic index, it is a fat. Limit fat servings to six per day.

- ◆ Chayote—This is a fruit, is high in nutrients, has no fat, and only contains 5 grams of carbs per cup. It would be considered a 0 glycemic index.

- ◆ Nuts and seeds—Serving size for these are 1 TB. seeds or 6 to 10 nuts. Even though these have a low to a 0 glycemic index and 1 or less glycemic load per serving, they are also fats. Limit fat servings to six per day.

So go ahead and eat these healthful vegetables and nuts. In the quantities recommended, they're packed with valuable nutrition, they don't raise your blood sugar levels, and they don't stimulate insulin overproduction.

Yes, your mother was right: You should eat your vegetables … especially these!

The Least You Need to Know

- ◆ Carbohydrates can be fattening or thinning, based on how you eat them.

- ◆ Pasta can be low-, medium-, or high-glycemic, based on how long you cook it.

- ◆ The more slowly a starch or sugar is digested, the lower its glycemic index.

- ◆ Processed foods are generally higher glycemic than their unprocessed counterparts.

- ◆ Some carbs, such as the nonstarchy vegetables that contain a very small quantity of carbs, have a glycemic index of 0, so they don't have any impact on your glycemic load.

Tallying Your Glycemic Load

In This Chapter

- Knowing quantity and quality
- Calculating glycemic load
- Eating acidic foods
- Determining the glycemic load for a recipe or a meal

One thing's for certain. Our bodies and how they process food are very complex. The old-time formula for weight loss, "eat less and exercise more," is just too simplistic.

The glycemic index is based on the complex, interrelated aspects of how our bodies process what we eat. Unfortunately, at first the glycemic index can seem complex, too. But don't be intimidated by it. It's fundamentally simple. And, as you learn more, you'll appreciate how brilliantly it aligns with how your body's digestion functions.

So let's explore the glycemic index a little deeper. In this chapter you learn how the amount of low-, medium- or high-glycemic carbohydrates you eat makes a difference in your weight-loss results. The way you account for quantity is by calculating the glycemic load.

Glyco Lingo

Glycemic load lets you predict what effect a serving of a carbohydrate food will have on your blood sugar levels.

Wrong Weigh

Because low-glycemic foods aid in satiety, it is harder to overeat with low-glycemic carbohydrate foods, but, not impossible. Eating too many low-glycemic carbohydrates can increase your overall glycemic load and slow or even halt your weight loss. Be sure you take into account the quantity of your food as well as the quality, to achieve your desired weight-loss goals.

Quantity and Quality

The *glycemic load* is the key to knowing how much of a carb to eat. As you have already learned, the glycemic index gives you information about the quality of a carbohydrate. The numerical value tells you how eating that carbohydrate will affect your blood sugar levels. The glycemic index alone, however, doesn't give you a guide for how much of any carbohydrate you can or should eat.

When the glycemic index first became popular, many people assumed that as long as a food was low-glycemic, it didn't matter how much of it we ate. Wrong. Indiscriminately filling up on too many carbohydrates, even low-glycemic carbs, can cause weight gain.

Yes, quantity makes a big difference, which means we need a simple way to calculate how to eat "glycemically smart" throughout the day. That's where the glycemic load comes in handy. It's a more explicit guide for how many carbohydrates to eat *and* how to eat a balanced low-glycemic diet.

Calculating Glycemic Load

Even though you won't need a pencil, paper, and calculator to compute the glycemic load of your meals, it's helpful to understand how glycemic load is calculated.

Body of Knowledge

New glycemic index tables include the glycemic load for average serving sizes. Until recently, the tables were calculated for countries such as Canada and Australia that measure food quantities in grams. This made it challenging for us in the United States to use glycemic load. Most of us don't know how to convert grams into ounces and then into cups and tablespoons. Fortunately, the glycemic index has become so popular that newer glycemic charts give quantities in more familiar measurements such as cups and ounces.

To calculate the glycemic load of a quantity of a carbohydrate, multiply the glycemic index value times the quantity of carbohydrates of the serving in grams, then divide by 100. The equation looks like this:

GI value × grams per serving / 100 = glycemic load

Here's an example of the difference in glycemic load between a five-ounce serving of baked white potato and a five-ounce serving of baked yams:

White potatoes:

5 ounces

34 grams carbohydrates

Glycemic index is 85 (high-glycemic)

Glycemic load is 29 or (34 × 85)/100

Yams:

5 ounces

34 grams carbohydrates

Glycemic index is 37 (low-glycemic)

Glycemic load is 13 or (34 × 37)/100

The glycemic load of white potatoes is twice that of the yams, so its effect on a person's blood sugar is twice as great as eating the yams. This is a very significant difference in terms of weight loss. Remember, you want to keep your insulin levels low and this is how you do it—by eating a low-glycemic load.

Thin-spiration _____

At a large family dinner, Lucy baked an equal amount of white potatoes and yams and put both in a bowl on the dinner table. She wanted to observe which ones her teenaged sons and their friends would eat. She didn't mention the nutritional or glycemic index value; in fact, she didn't say anything about them at all.

As she cleared the table, she observed that all the yams had been eaten while plenty of white baked potatoes remained. Seems the teens thought the baked yams were more appetizing. Most likely, you will, too.

Let's look at another example, this time with dessert.

Tofu-based frozen dessert, chocolate, sweetened with high-fructose corn syrup:

$^1/_2$ cup

30 carbohydrate grams

Glycemic index is 115

Glycemic load is 34

Premium ice cream:

$^1/_2$ cup

15 carbohydrate grams

Glycemic index is 37

Glycemic load is 5.

Glyco Lingo

A **trigger food** is one that can lead you to overeating—or even to binge eating. Some common trigger foods are candy, chips, popcorn, donuts, and ice cream. If you have a trigger food and find it impossible to eat only a small amount, it's best not to eat it at all.

Yes, a half cup of absolutely rich and luscious premium ice cream has a glycemic load of only 5. The supposed "healthy" Tofutti has a load of 34.

So which is healthier for your heart, your insulin levels, insulin resistance, and more? The correct answer is the premium ice cream, provided that you eat no more than $^1/_2$ cup and the amount of saturated fat is within your limits for that day. Isn't this great? If ice cream is not a *trigger food* for you, you can have some ice cream and lose weight, too.

High, Medium, and Low Loads

By now you're familiar with how individual carbohydrates are classified based on their glycemic index value: high, 70 and over; medium, 56 to 69; and low, 55 or lower.

Now we need to introduce you to how carbohydrate portions are categorized based on the glycemic load.

A glycemic load of 20 or above is high, 11 to 19 is medium, and 10 or below is low. The serving of yams in the previous example is medium while the serving of white potatoes is high. The glycemic load of the Tofutti is high and the ice cream is low.

As a review, to calculate glycemic load (GL), both the grams of carbohydrates and the glycemic index are put into the calculation. GL = carbohydrate grams × glycemic index divided by 100. If a very small amount of a high-glycemic food is eaten, it does not have a big impact. However, research indicates that the more frequently you eat high-glycemic foods, such as the Tofutti, the more likely you are to experience adverse health and weight gain. The reason for this appears to be that the higher-glycemic foods do not satisfy hunger as well as the low-glycemic foods do. So in practice, it's better to eat mostly low-glycemic foods and only eat high-glycemic items sparingly, if at all. In this comparison, you'd be better off choosing the ice cream. Your waistline will celebrate—or at least be smaller.

Your Daily Allotment

The key to success with glycemic index weight loss is simple: Eat within your glycemic load allotment every day. Here are some guidelines for choosing your allotment. Start with these recommendations and then modify them if necessary. You may need to lower them if you aren't losing weight, or raise them if you are losing too quickly.

◆ Start with a glycemic load allotment of 60 to 75 per day, making sure to spread this out over the course of the day. You might have 15 at each meal and three snacks of about 10 each.

Body of Knowledge

If you don't want to calculate the glycemic load, you can count carbs. To start, allow 30 grams of low-glycemic carbohydrates per meal and 10 to 30 grams of low-glycemic carbohydrates for snacks. Eat three meals and two to three snacks. Eat only low glycemic carbohydrates (the two bottom tiers of the new Food Guide Pyramid). Count all carbohydrates, even the nonstarchy "free food" vegetables. The total grams of carbohydrates for the entire day with meals and snacks should be less than 150. Some people may need to keep their carb total between 90 to 120 to lose weight.

◆ If you are pregnant or nursing, you'll need to increase your glycemic load to as much as 130 per day. It is not recommended to lose weight while you are pregnant or in the first four months of nursing.

◆ A highly active woman or a male may need to eat a glycemic load of between 100 to 150 to give them plenty of energy.

◆ A younger person needs to eat a higher glycemic load than a person who is older, because metabolism slows with age.

Wrong Weigh

Don't save up your glycemic load allotment and eat it all at one meal. You won't be able to lose weight if you do. Instead, you'll be triggering your body's fat-storing system with a rapid increase in blood sugar and insulin levels.

◆ A person with a lower percentage of body fat can eat a higher daily allotment than a person with a high body fat percentage.

Start with the previous recommendations. After several weeks, you'll learn how the different carbohydrates work in your body. And if you aren't losing weight, lower your glycemic allotment to a 50 to 60 glycemic load until you are losing weight and your clothes fit looser. It is not healthy for most of us to go lower than a 50 glycemic load.

Wrong Weigh

Janice found what she thought was a great way to get her five servings of vegetables and fruits every day. For lunch, she made a smoothie of a banana, a cup of fruit juice, strawberries, cherries, and pineapple. She added some yogurt and ice and voilà! She was obtaining all her necessary antioxidants, vitamins, and fiber in one single meal. Plus she didn't need to mess with any more vegetables or fruit the rest of the day. Whoa. Just a minute. The glycemic load of that smoothie was off the charts. Not only that, somehow she missed the vegetable part of the government's recommendations. No wonder she wasn't losing weight but, rather, gaining it.

Combination Foods

The glycemic index and the glycemic load work very well for individual foods. So far, so good. But what if you want to fix your favorite recipe? How can you figure out the glycemic index or the glycemic load?

In a scientific sense, you can't calculate the glycemic index of a combination of ingredients. The very fact of the combination changes the value. For example, pizza is a very complex food. The crust is made of white or whole-wheat bread, which will make it high-glycemic. The tomato sauce is medium-glycemic. The meats and cheeses in the topping are zero, as they contain virtually no carbs. If you intuitively average the glycemic indexes, you'd guess that pizza is medium-glycemic. But, actually, pizza is usually low-glycemic with a glycemic load of about nine per slice.

Let's look at the factors that contribute to this surprising result:

◆ The starch, in this case the flour, is enriched and in very fine particles, so the starch is easily digested, making it high-glycemic.

◆ Pizza is a high-fat food. Fat slows down digestion, so the starch isn't as quickly digested as if the bread were eaten alone.

◆ Tomatoes are acidic, as are some of the possible toppings, such as olives, peppers, and pepperoni. Acid slows down the digestion of starch.

Now, here's the problem. Although pizza is a low-glycemic food, beware. Eat it sparingly, if at all. Here's why. Pizza bread is high-glycemic and you don't want to load up on high-glycemic foods, even if they are balanced with acid and fat. Plus, it's important to keep your saturated fat at about 10 percent of your daily food intake, which is really hard to do when you eat more than a small piece of pizza. So one slice of pizza now and then—say once a week—is fine. Be sure to add a fresh green salad with vinegar and oil dressing to add fiber and an acid food to the meal.

Wrong Weigh

One of the big weight-loss challenges with foods such as pizza, cookies, and donuts is that it's hard to stop with just one. Even though some could be low- or medium-glycemic because they contain eggs and fat, they can still ruin your weight-loss efforts if you eat more than a small amount. Eat only one slice of pizza or one cookie or even just a half so that you gain taste satisfaction but not pounds. Or better yet, in the case of pizza, eat the topping and hold the crust. Overeating is always fattening—it increases insulin resistance.

Calculations for Meals and Recipes

You can calculate the glycemic index and glycemic load for recipes and meals. Joan did this for every recipe in our cookbook *The Complete Idiot's Guide to Terrific Diabetic Meals.* However, we don't recommend you do these calculations on a day-to-day basis unless you love arithmetic, calculators, doing ratios, and other aspects of mathematics.

Here's how to calculate the glycemic index of a recipe. The result of your calculation will be an estimate only. The only way to know the exact glycemic index is to test it on volunteers in a research setting. But we find an estimate to be just fine for everyday eating.

Step 1: List all carbohydrate ingredients and the amount of carbohydrates for each ingredient. List all ingredients whether or not they contain carbohydrates.

Step 2: Add the total of carbohydrates to determine how many carbs are in the recipe or meal.

Step 3: By doing ratios, determine what percentage of the total carbs comes from each ingredient.

Step 4: Multiply the percentage of each ingredient by its glycemic index value.

Step 5: Add all the values from step 4 together. This is the calculated glycemic index of the recipe or meal.

Here's how to calculate the glycemic load of a serving for a meal or recipe.

Step 1: Start with the calculated glycemic index of the recipes or meals from step 5.

Step 2: Multiply by the total number of grams of carbohydrates in the recipe or meal.

Step 3: Divide the number in step 2 by the number of servings in the recipe.

Step 4: Divide the number by 100. That's the glycemic load.

Body of Knowledge

Doing the calculations for the glycemic load of combination foods, such as recipes and meals, can't give you a truly accurate answer, but you can get close. The glycemic index of a food can vary based on where it's grown, how long it ripened, and the kind of soil in which it was grown. Also, when ingredients are cooked together, the glycemic index changes. But because eating isn't an exact science anyway, getting close can provide you with valuable and useful information.

Example:

Chicken Broccoli and Pasta with Slivered Almonds

Serves 2

Serving size: 2 cups

Ingredients	Carb Grams	Percentage	Glycemic Index
Broccoli 2 cups	10	.22	0
Red pepper 1 cup	5	.11	0
Whole wheat pasta ⅔ cup	30	.66	32
Olive oil 1 tsp.	0	0	0
Chicken 6 oz.	0	0	0
Sliced almonds 2 TB.	2	.04	0
Totals	47		21 (.66 × 32 = 21)

21 is the GI for the recipe. To calculate GL for this example, because it contains 2 servings, it is:

$$47 \times 21 / 2 = 10.5$$

10.5 is the GL per serving. To determine the GL per serving:

$$\frac{GI \times carb/serving}{100} \quad or \quad \frac{21 \times 23 = 4.83 \text{ or } 5.}{100}$$

For this recipe, 5 is the GL and 21 is the GI.

The above calculations don't account for some ingredients that could lower the effective glycemic index and glycemic load. Fats, proteins, and acids can change the result. As of now, there's no way to predict how much these kinds of ingredients would change your results. That's why the above is only an estimate.

Possible Discrepancies

The glycemic index is a scientific development and, as such, it isn't developed all the way. There are some things we don't yet know for sure:

◆ How much the fats in a meal lower the effective glycemic index

◆ Why cinnamon lowers the glycemic effect of a meal

◆ How to predict the effect that protein has on blood sugar when eaten with a carbohydrate and fat

◆ How much a high-stress life can change the effective glycemic index and glycemic load of a meal

◆ How a carbohydrate of starch reacts in the body versus the way a carbohydrate of fruit does. The underlying assumption in the glycemic index theory is that they react in the same way but this is still not verified as scientifically correct.

◆ How to predict individual variations

Stayed tuned to learn more about the glycemic index as more information becomes available.

The Least You Need to Know

◆ The quantity of carbohydrates you eat is measured by the glycemic load.

◆ Acid-based foods can lower the glycemic load of a meal by one third.

◆ You can calculate the glycemic index and load of a recipe and a meal.

◆ The glycemic index is still being researched, so stay tuned as we learn more about this wonderful weight-loss tool.

Part 2

Designing Your Glycemic Index Weight-Loss Program

You'll begin your program by learning how to keep your metabolism high and progress to choosing one of two glycemic index weight-loss programs, either the Keep It Simple or the Comprehensive program. You'll be able to stay the course using the power of your mind coupled with affirmations to visualize yourself at your ideal size.

Your maintenance program is the same as your weight-loss program, but you'll be eating more medium- and high-glycemic carbohydrates. As you attain your ideal size, you'll feel so good and have so much energy to burn that you'll find yourself falling in love with this healthful way of eating.

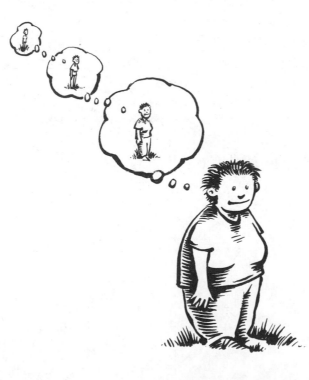

Chapter 6

Keeping Your Metabolism High

In This Chapter

- ◆ Understanding metabolic resistance
- ◆ Boosting your metabolism
- ◆ Using low-glycemic eating to lift the basal metabolic rate
- ◆ Correcting slow metabolism

Perhaps you've thought something like this as the pounds have crept on: "If only my metabolism were higher, I never would have gained all this weight in the first place. I would be able to eat whatever I wanted, whenever I wanted, and never gain a pound."

Unfortunately, this is wishful thinking. Very few people can eat anything at any time and maintain a healthy weight for life. However, there is some truth to the notion that your weight is dependent on your metabolism. Your basal metabolic rate plays a major role in your glycemic index weight-loss success.

Decreasing body fat is only one method for increasing your basal metabolic rate. In this chapter, you learn more ways to increase your metabolism during your glycemic index weight-loss program and throughout your lifelong maintenance program.

What's Slowing Your Metabolism?

Although some people can keep their metabolism high throughout their lives, most can't. Certain biological factors are, well, facts of life. After a person's biological prime, say at about age 30 or 35, the body's hormonal system begins to slow down and continues slowing down with every passing decade. As hormone production slows, so, too, does the *basal metabolic rate.*

With a slower metabolism, the body naturally increases fat storage while slowing down the production of muscle mass. As a person gains more body fat, metabolism slows down further, creating a cycle that keeps metabolism low and fat storage high. The reason your body does this is because it takes more energy, or calories, to maintain a pound of muscle than a pound of fat. So if we compare two women who are the same height, weight, and age, the woman who has a body fat percentage of 25 percent will typically have a higher metabolism than the woman who has a body fat percentage of 35 percent. Quite simply, lower body fat percentage translates into a higher metabolism. So one goal for increasing your metabolism is to increase your muscle mass and decrease your body fat percentage.

Glyco Lingo

Basal metabolic rate is the rate at which a person's body uses energy in a relaxed state. The body really does "burn" through food, actually producing heat and providing energy to your organs and muscles. (Sometimes it is referred to as the thermic or thermogenic effect of your body.)

A diet high in carbohydrates—especially one high in high-glycemic carbohydrates—increases insulin levels. Excess insulin stores excess blood sugar as fat. Too much insulin increases a person's fat stores and body fat percentage, eventually slowing metabolism.

Fortunately, the opposite is also true. When you eat the low-glycemic way, your body produces less insulin. When insulin levels are low, your body isn't storing fat. A low-glycemic weight-loss program uses up its own stored fat for energy, so your body fat percentage drops, your metabolism rises, and you lose weight!

Metabolic Resistance

Some people have such slow metabolisms that losing weight is very difficult. These people have *metabolic resistance*. This is often caused by having too high of a body fat percentage, but it can also be caused by other factors that include decreased mobility, genetic predisposition to insulin resistance, hormonal imbalances due to medications, poor sleep, and stress. Ideal body fat percentages are as follows:

Women:	Up to age 20	14% to 21%
	Ages 20 to 50	17% to 27%
	Age 50+	20% to 30%
Men:	Up to age 20	9% to 15%
	Ages 20 to 50	14% to 21%
	Age 50+	19% to 23%

Within these ranges, your metabolism is working at top performance and you won't be considered overweight. Use this chart to set your desired body fat percentage. You can have your current body fat percentage measured at a health club or fitness center. There are many ways to measure body fat, including bio-impedance, near-infrared interactance, dual-energy x-ray absorptionmetry, underwater body measuring, MRI (Magnetic Resonance Imaging), CT (Computerized Tomography), and body composition by air displacement. The important thing is to consistently use the same method on a regular basis. That way you'll get a more reliable measure of progress.

A person can also become metabolically resistant to weight loss because of many years of yo-yo dieting. Yo-yo dieting causes the body to increase fat storage because insulin levels could remain high both during the weight-loss times and the weight-gain times. Remember, not all diet programs keep insulin levels low. In fact, many don't; so a person could lose pounds and still gain fat.

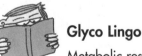

Glyco Lingo

Metabolic resistance is a condition in which a person's basal metabolic rate is so low that the person has a difficult time losing weight.

Another factor that can contribute to metabolic resistance is leading a sedentary lifestyle. The couch and the office chair in front of the computer are your enemies! The more you move, the easier it is to lose weight. If you suspect that you're metabolically resistant to weight loss, be sure to include exercise, both strength training and aerobics, with a low-glycemic weight-loss program.

Boosting Your Metabolism

Nothing can be done about your age, so don't worry about it. You simply are the age you are, and yes, your metabolism slows down accordingly. But all is not lost. You can rev up your metabolism in spite of your age, no matter what age you are. Here's what to do beyond eating the low-glycemic way.

Avoid Overeating

Low-glycemic weight loss only works to the extent that you don't overeat. When you overeat, your body's insulin levels become elevated and your body starts storing fat.

When low-carb diets, as opposed to low-glycemic weight-loss programs, first became popular in the 1970s, many well-intentioned experts believed that individuals could eat as much fat and meat as they wanted, provided they avoided most carbohydrates. Think Atkins. What we know today, 20 years later, is that it's not healthy or a good idea to overdo any food. Too much fat or too much protein is not advisable. Besides the fact that the calorie count is too high for healthful weight loss, huge amounts of fat or protein threaten your overall health. Even eating too many low-glycemic carbohydrates is not a good idea. The good news is that it is much harder to overeat when eating low-glycemic carbohydrates. You will find eating low-glycemic to be very satisfying and it will help with satiety.

Your unstretched stomach is about the size of your fist. So make a fist right now and take a look at the volume we're talking about. Your body needs about that much food three or four times a day. If you eat much more than that at a sitting, you're overeating, and you're slowing down your metabolism in the process.

Increase Muscle Mass

Your metabolism increases with an increase in muscle mass, so it's time to start an enthusiastic program for strength training. No matter what your age, you can produce really fast and satisfying results when you pick up those weights and pump.

You can pump iron at a fitness center or a health club. Use the machines, use the free weights, or participate in some version of a "power-pump" fitness class. If you prefer a more serene environment, do your strength training with a Pilates class or a home video. You'll soon look as if you've lost weight, your clothes will fit better, and you'll lose weight faster.

Enjoy Your ZZZs

You need an adequate amount of sleep every night for your metabolism to run at optimal speed. Be sure you don't try to shortcut your sleep. No one is going to give you a badge of honor for sleeping fewer hours than your body requires. But you may inhibit your ability to lose weight if you don't sleep enough.

When you don't get enough sleep on a regular basis, your body's stress hormones, adrenaline and cortisol, increase. With an increase in stress hormones comes an increase in insulin levels. That means your body starts storing fat, which in turn slows down your metabolism. A vicious cycle.

Balance Your Eating

Your body responds best when you eat balanced meals that contain protein, fat, and carbohydrates. When you're eating the low-glycemic way, carbs are still an important and essential part of your meals. Don't totally exclude them. You could stall your metabolism. If you eat out-of-balance meals once in while, don't worry; you can make up for it at the next meal. But if you avoid all carbs, all fats, or all protein repeatedly for a week or two, your body won't receive the nutrition it needs.

> ### Body of Knowledge
>
> An easy way to determine how much sleep you need is to go to bed earlier and avoid setting your alarm clock. Instead, wake up naturally and note how long you slept. You need to do this every day for about a week to get a clear answer. For practical reasons, you might need to try this experiment during a vacation. After you've learned your natural sleep amount, schedule your life so that you get the ZZZs you need.

In addition, it's important to spread out the food that you eat somewhat evenly throughout your day. Research shows that skipping meals increases your chance of becoming overweight.

When you're deprived of proper nutrition, your body starts behaving as if it's in a famine situation and slows its metabolism; plus it starts storing fat. From the body's perspective, the advantage of slowing metabolism during a famine is to ensure that you have enough fuel on which to live. Fat has more energy per pound than muscle, so fat becomes an ideal fuel source.

Avoid High-Glycemic Foods

By eating starchy and sugary high-glycemic foods, you increase insulin levels and encourage your body to store fat. As you proceed with low-glycemic weight loss, you'll learn exactly what glycemic load your body can handle without gaining weight.

Perhaps you'll eat high-glycemic foods once in a while, but most likely, cookies and candy won't be a large part of your maintenance plan. It's impossible to tell you how much high-glycemic food your body can handle, because everyone's needs are different. But one thing is certain: Your metabolism will be higher if you avoid them.

Drink Caffeine Cautiously

How caffeine affects your weight loss can vary. Some people can continue to drink a couple of cups of coffee or a caffeinated beverage every day and have great success on a low-glycemic weight-loss program. Others may find that it slows down progress.

Caffeine all by itself, even without cream and sugar, can stimulate the production of insulin because it can indirectly raise blood glucose levels by stimulating the release of glycogen stores. And, as stated previously, this can increase fat storage and thwart fat burning.

The only way to determine how caffeine works for you is to stop drinking it for a week or so and notice if your weight loss increases. If you hit a weight-loss plateau, try eliminating caffeine. That might be enough to move you off the plateau.

Caffeine is in coffee and black and green teas, as well as in many soft drinks, both naturally and artificially sweetened.

Fewer Sweet Sips

Sipping on sweet-tasting beverages frequently can forestall weight loss. These include both naturally and artificially sweetened drinks. Additionally, avoiding artificially sweetened drinks such as "diet" sodas will help break the habit of longing for a sweet taste in your mouth.

One theory suggests that when your body tastes something sweet, it makes the assumption that food is on the way. For some biological reason not yet fully understood, your body thinks it's time to store fat. So enjoy your sweet-tasting beverages with a meal or all by themselves, but avoid sipping on them frequently all day long. Instead, sip on water. It's an all-time winner.

Calcium Intake

In studies, calcium has been shown to assist with weight loss, so make sure you eat plenty of foods that contain this bone-building nutrient. Calcium is found in low-carb foods including salmon with bones, sardines, seafood, and broccoli, asparagus, almonds, cabbage, and dark-green, leafy vegetables. Other foods that provide calcium include milk, yogurt, and cheese. The good news is that you'll be eating plenty of calcium-rich vegetables and lower-fat dairy products on your low-glycemic weight-loss program. You'll learn more about dairy in Chapter 13.

Taking a calcium supplement may also be helpful. The adult body needs between 1000 to 1500 mg of calcium a day.

Alcoholic Beverages

For the purposes of your glycemic index weight-loss program, alcohol is a food, contains calories, and needs to be noted in your daily food journal. A 3.5 ounce glass of white wine has 70 calories and one gram of carbohydrates. Just one ounce of 90-proof liquor has 73 calories and no carbs. And 12 ounces of beer has 146 calories and 13 grams of carbs.

The glycemic index of alcoholic beverages hasn't been tested with any accuracy because the glycemic index changes based on when the alcohol is consumed—before, during, or after a meal. We do know that alcohol can increase and then lower blood sugar levels, making them hard to predict. However, with all alcoholic beverages, even low-glycemic alcoholic beverages, you need to be cautious. The body uses alcohol as fuel first, and only after the alcohol is used up does it obtain energy from your fat stores. This means that enjoying a glass or two of wine with dinner will stall your fat-burning process.

Thin-spiration

Alcoholic beverages can stimulate production of the stress hormone cortisol. How much varies by frequency, amount, and of course, by person. High levels of cortisol are known to help pack on weight around your middle. They don't call 'em beer bellies for nothing.

Wrong Weigh

You can now purchase low-carb beer, but should you? Probably not. Low-carb beer still contains alcohol, which can elevate cortisol levels and insulin levels, while stimulating appetite. You'll drink fewer carbs than with regular beer, but you'll still need to contend with the fattening and appetite-stimulating qualities in beer.

Another consideration is that alcohol is an appetite stimulant. Research shows that its effects vary with different people. Some people never notice an increase in appetite. Others notice an increased appetite effect for up to one week after that single glass of wine, which is exactly what you don't want.

The way to determine how alcohol affects your body is to keep a record of all the foods you eat and drink, including alcoholic ones. Review your records for the week after you drank an alcoholic beverage. If you ate more food than normal for the next several days, alcohol could be an appetite stimulant for you. If a glass of wine stalls your progress or stimulates your appetite too much, pass on the alcohol in the future. Of course, it's safest to simply avoid alcoholic beverages altogether during your weight-loss program.

Eat

If you are hungry and it's time for a meal or snack, go ahead and, by all means, eat. Don't skip meals thinking that it will help you lose weight. Skipping meals when you're hungry can actually slow down your metabolism, because your body starts to use muscle tissue instead of fat for energy. So keep on eating regularly to keep your metabolism stoked.

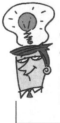

Thin-spiration

One fabulous advantage of low-glycemic weight loss is that you are supposed to eat meals and snacks. You don't skip meals. You don't rely on liquid meals. And unlike diets that simply restrict calories without regard to food type, following a low-glycemic plan allows you to eat plenty of delicious foods and continue to lose weight.

Weight-Loss Blockers

Before you embark on your low-glycemic weight-loss program, you need to know that some medical conditions could prevent or stall your progress. If any of these apply to you, be sure to check with your doctor for advice.

Medications

Some prescription and over-the-counter medications can prevent or stall weight loss. They increase a person's metabolic resistance. These include the following:

◆ Steroids such as prednisone and, to a lesser degree, asthma inhalers

◆ Some anticonvulsants

◆ Some antidepressants

◆ Some hormone-replacement therapy drugs

◆ Some birth control pills

◆ Insulin and insulin-stimulating drugs

Not all drugs in the previous categories work the same way. If you suspect that your medication is thwarting your weight-loss efforts, talk with your doctor or pharmacist about other options. Discuss alternative choices, such as using nutritional supplements or lifestyle changes, to help you eliminate the need for these medications.

As you experience success with your glycemic index weight-loss program, your need for some medications, such as those for high blood pressure, may decrease or be eliminated.

Yeast Infections

Chronic Candida albicans, or yeast infections, can prevent weight loss. Everyone's body contains both beneficial bacteria and yeast. It's only when the balance between the two is disrupted that a person's yeast overgrows to the point of a yeast infection. Yeast infections include such symptoms as rashes that itch, vaginitis, ringworm, athlete's foot, thrush, nail infections, and jock itch.

Yeast overgrowth can increase appetite, especially for sweets and high-glycemic carbs, which can result in weight gain. Those food cravings make it hard to follow a weight-loss program.

Often yeast infections are caused by the overuse of antibiotics, which have destroyed all the body's beneficial bacteria. Eliminating a yeast infection will help you lose weight. Many natural solutions can work. Try these suggestions:

◆ Take an acidophilus supplement that contains bifidobacterium and bulgaricus. If you are sensitive to dairy, use a supplement that doesn't contain milk cultures. Take as directed.

Glyco Lingo

An **alkaline–ash effect** occurs when the urine turns more alkaline. When the body is slightly alkaline, it's easier for it to maintain the proper bacteria-yeast balance level so that a person can reduce or eliminate urinary tract infections as well as yeast infections. You can test your urine pH with litmus strips available at pharmacies.

◆ Mix up a powdered "greens" drink in water twice a day and drink. The drink can help produce an *alkaline-ash effect* and is filled with an abundance of beneficial phytonutrients, minerals, and vitamins. Yeast flourishes in an acidic environment, so by making the body slightly alkaline, the yeast dies off. Nutritionists frequently advocate that having a slightly alkaline body is healthier. You'll find "greens" drink mixes at the health food store.

You can find other solutions for yeast infections at health-food stores. And if these suggestions don't work for you, you can also contact your health-care provider.

Low Thyroid

Your thyroid gland regulates your metabolism. If it's not functioning correctly, you could have metabolic resistance to weight loss due to a low thyroid. Other symptoms include lethargy and fatigue, depression, sensitivity to cold, dry skin, chronic constipation, hair loss, poor memory, or elevated cholesterol levels.

If you suspect you have an under-functioning thyroid, ask your doctor for a thyroid test to evaluate your T3, T4, and TSH levels. If they're low, you may need a prescription for a thyroid hormone.

The Least You Need to Know

◆ Metabolic resistance is corrected through low-glycemic eating and lifestyle changes.

◆ Use strength training and aerobic exercise as ways to boost your basal metabolic rate.

◆ Increase your overall daily activity level.

◆ Make sure you get a good night's sleep most nights to keep your metabolism high.

◆ A low thyroid hormone, yeast overgrowth, and some medications can stall or prevent weight loss.

The New Food Pyramid

In This Chapter

- ◆ Reviewing the Old Food Pyramid
- ◆ Creating the New Food Pyramid
- ◆ Learning the Glycemic Index Food Pyramid
- ◆ Using the Plate Method

As you read this book, you've noticed that food and eating "ain't what they used to be." Today, our knowledge about food and how it works in the body is different from even 10 years ago.

Remember when you were taught about food and eating in elementary school? The chart on the wall was the Traditional Food Pyramid and it recommended that a person eat 5 to 11 servings of food made from grains, such as bread or cereal, every day. The traditional pyramid does not differentiate between processed and unprocessed grains, types of fats, or types of protein foods. Because much of our food in the United States is processed, many of us eat 6 to 11 servings of processed grain foods, instead of whole, coarse, unprocessed types of grain foods. These processed foods, such as white breads and instant cereals, are very high-glycemic and can cause weight gain. No wonder more than 67 percent of the adult population in the United States is overweight or obese! Eating that many servings of high-glycemic foods will not help a person lose weight.

It's time to update the food pyramid. In this chapter, you learn about the problems with the Old Food Pyramid and become familiar with an improved food pyramid that reflects our new knowledge about the glycemic index. You also learn about the Plate Method of serving yourself.

The Traditional Food Pyramid

The purpose of any food pyramid is to help plan meals and to provide guidelines for a healthy diet. Basically, foods at the top of the pyramid should be eaten the least; those at the bottom should be eaten the most. The food pyramid now widely used by dietitians and nutritionists was designed in 1992. We'll call it the Old Food Pyramid. It needs updating, but let's take a closer look at it anyway. You'll recognize it as the one you learned about in school and be able to understand why it is incorrect.

At the top of the Old Food Pyramid are fats, oils, and sweets, recommending that these be eaten sparingly.

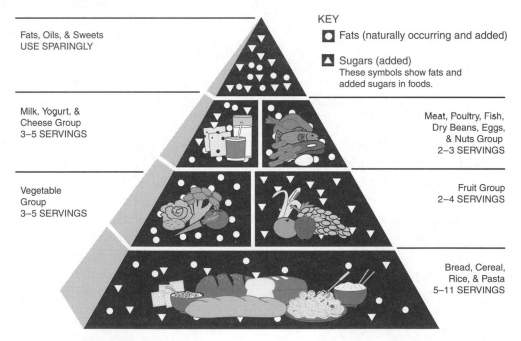

The Old Food Pyramid.

The next tier down includes dairy products, such as milk, yogurt, and cheese. Recommendation: Eat 3 to 5 servings a day. Alongside dairy are meats, including poultry, fish, eggs, and nuts. (No, nuts and eggs aren't "meats" but they fall into this category nonetheless.) Recommendation: Eat 2 to 3 servings a day.

The next level down includes fruits (Recommendation: 2 to 4 servings a day) and vegetables (Recommendation: 3 to 5 servings a day).

So far, so good. This pyramid is somewhat consistent with a healthy low-glycemic diet and includes a nice emphasis on fruits and vegetables. The problem comes with the bottom level. There you'll find starches, breads, cereals, rice, and grains. The Old Food Pyramid recommends eating 5 to 11 servings a day, and does not specify eating the unprocessed whole types of grains, but, rather depicts photos of more highly processed types of starches.

Don't do it. The Old Food Pyramid recommends eating so much of the starchy high-glycemic foods, that for most of us, this could aggravate problems with insulin resistance.

Thin-spiration

Now that you are re-educating yourself about the foods that help you lose weight and the ones that can cause fat storage, be sure to let others know what works. Tell your doctor, the school nurse, your healthcare practitioners, and by all means, teach your children to eat based on the glycemic index. Teach them about the New Food Pyramid.

Development in Progress

The USDA (United States Department of Agriculture) is aware that the current food pyramid no longer works. That much is good. They're attempting to revise it. This is also good. And they're seeking input from lots of sources. Some of this is good and some is questionable.

We applaud that some of the input is coming from independent research sources. But some of it is coming from food lobbying groups and food processors' trade associations. Unfortunately, much of their information is based on research studies paid for by special interest groups, such as the American Dairy Council and the Bakers Association.

The foods that work best in your body aren't determined by special interest group lobbying. Your body doesn't care what they think or how they make money. What your body needs—to be healthy and stay at an ideal size—has nothing to do with politics and a whole lot to do with your biology and your DNA. We hope that valid scientific research about foods will take precedence over food-industry paid research.

The end results based on government recommendations have yet to be published. In the meantime, several health and medical organizations have designed new food pyramids in an effort to best educate their patients.

> ### Body of Knowledge
>
> It isn't surprising that the new Food Guide Pyramid was developed both for persons with diabetes and for people who want to lose weight. Both groups need to keep their blood sugar levels low. For people who want to lose weight, this helps prevent the body from storing fat and reduces the likelihood of insulin resistance, which can also cause weight gain.

> ### Wrong Weigh
>
> When referring to the Food Guide Pyramid, remember to be careful about your serving sizes. Too much food is still too much food, even if it's low-glycemic. A great rule of thumb is to never, never, never overeat. As you read earlier in this book, overeating leads to insulin resistance.

Glycemic Index Food Pyramid

A new food pyramid based on glycemic index research has been developed by two health-care practitioners at the University of Utah Diabetes Center. Dana Clarke, M.D., CDE, and Joan Clark, MS, RD, CDE, and coauthor of this book, have developed a new food pyramid that's based on research on the glycemic index. It's called the Food Guide Pyramid for Type 2 Diabetes and Weight Management.

This food pyramid supports you in losing weight. Refer to this and you can't go wrong in making your food selections.

At the top of the Food Guide Pyramid are the foods to eat sparingly and infrequently. These are high-glycemic carbohydrates that have little to no nutritional value, such as syrup, sweets, and baked goods that have a glycemic index value of 72 or above.

The next level down includes high-glycemic carbohydrates that have some nutritional value. The list includes some breakfast cereals and sticky white rice. You can eat up to two servings a day, but on your glycemic index weight-loss program, it's best to eat only one serving or none at all. A serving size is $^1/_2$ cup.

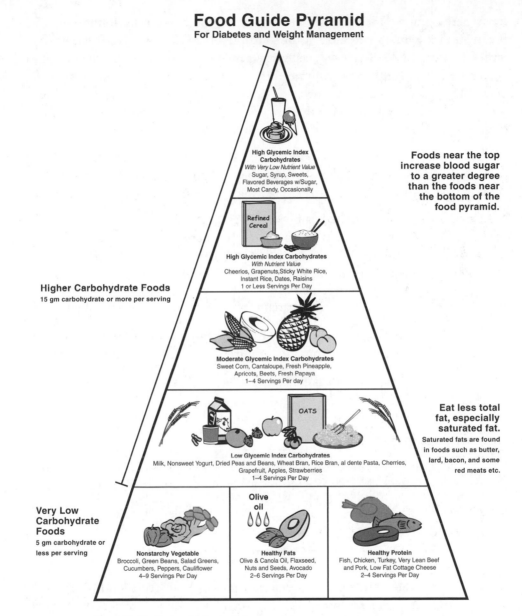

Food Guide Pyramid for weight management.

Next are moderate-glycemic carbohydrates such as apricots, papayas, fresh pineapple, and raisins. You can eat 2 to 4 servings a day, but for weight loss eat 1 to 2 servings if any at all. A serving size is ½ cup.

From here on down through the pyramid are the foods you want to focus on eating for the best weight-loss results. At the fourth level are the low-glycemic carbohydrates. They include dairy products, such as milk, nonsweetened yogurt, legumes, 100 percent whole-wheat kernels, and rice bran, yams, sweet potatoes, and pasta cooked al dente. This level also includes lower-glycemic fruits, such as pears, apples, dates, oranges, cherries, and all others that are low-glycemic. A serving size is ¹/₂ cup. You can eat 1 to 4 servings per day of foods from level four.

At the bottom of the Food Guide Pyramid, level 5, are low carbohydrate foods. First, there are nonstarchy vegetables, such as broccoli, spinach, green beans, carrots, and asparagus. Eat 4 to 9 servings a day. A serving size is ¹/₂ cup cooked or one cup raw.

Next to the vegetables are the healthy fats, such as avocados, olive oil, nuts, and seeds. Eat 2 to 6 servings a day. Serving sizes vary here. For an avocado, use ¹/₄ small avocado; for nuts and seeds, six nuts or two tablespoons nuts and seeds; for oils and fats, one serving is one teaspoon.

The last item on the bottom level is healthy protein, including lean meats, seafood, poultry, and low-fat cottage cheese. Have 2 to 4 servings per day. A serving size is 3 to 4 ounces or ³/₄ cup cottage cheese. So to lose weight, eat mostly from the two lowest levels of the Food Guide Pyramid. Eat infrequently from the upper three levels.

By using this food guide, losing weight based on the glycemic index is easy. You can't go wrong eating foods in moderate serving sizes from the bottom two levels.

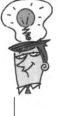

Thin-spiration _____

You may be wondering if your appetite can be satisfied by eating foods from the bottom two levels of the Food Guide Pyramid. Because lower-glycemic foods generally stay in your stomach longer, are generally more bulky, and help to keep blood sugar levels more stable, eating this way helps with satiety. We think you'll be pleasantly surprised. And your clothes will fit better.

Also remember that you don't need to totally give up your treat foods, just eat them very sparingly. As you start low-glycemic eating, however, you may benefit more to get rid of the "goodies" if they have been trigger foods for you in the past. Trigger foods tend to be psychologically addictive (the foods that cause you to keep going back for more and more servings). After eating this way for a while, many people find they actually crave salads and vegetables more than they desire the high-glycemic and fattening goodies.

So where do eggs fit in? Eggs are at the bottom of the food guide pyramid with the healthy protein. A serving is two eggs, or one egg and two egg whites, or 3 to 4 egg whites. If you are healthy and don't have heart disease or diabetes, you can eat whole eggs. But if you need to limit your dietary cholesterol or fat intake, then opt for egg whites instead. One egg equals seven grams of protein and five grams of fat. Egg whites do not contain fat, only protein, so eating these more often is not a problem.

The information and research on the glycemic index is ongoing, so look for new and updated information on glycemic index listings and food pyramids on the Internet and in newspapers and magazines.

Thin-spiration

Take the Food Guide Pyramid with you to the grocery store. Purchase foods in the bottom three levels, with an emphasis on the bottom two and you'll have the foods you need to be successful with glycemic index weight loss.

Sizing Up Your Plate

Another way to monitor your low-glycemic eating is by the Plate Method. This is especially helpful if you're a visual person and have been known to eat based on what your eyes can take in rather than on what your stomach can accommodate.

The Plate Method.

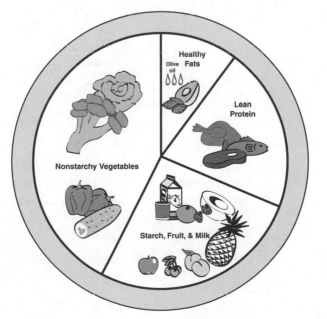

Wrong Weigh _____

Compare the size of a modern dinner plate to one in Grandma's china set. A modern dinner plate has 36 square inches of surface area, compared to 33 on Grandma's. Simply by using a smaller-sized plate, you'd eat less food at every meal. Eating all the food those extra three square inches can accommodate three times a day can add up quickly and add at least three more inches to your waistline.

The Plate Method is based on the glycemic index and takes into account what you need to eat to lose weight. So here's what to put on your plate:

◆ Fill just about half of your plate with nonstarchy vegetables. These include all nonstarchy vegetables located on the bottom of the pyramid. Except for beets, all nonstarchy vegetables are considered low-glycemic.

◆ Fill about one quarter of your plate with low-glycemic starches, fruit, or dairy products.

Body of Knowledge

By filling almost half your plate with vegetables and having another quarter for fruit, you'll be sure to eat the recommended amount of 5 to 10 servings of vegetables and fruit every day.

◆ One third of your plate is for lean protein, including meats, seafood, or poultry. Figure one third to be approximately 3 to 4 ounces.

◆ The remaining wedge of your plate, or about one eighth, is for healthy fats, such as olive oil, avocados, and nuts and seeds.

In actuality, your plate won't look exactly like this. Usually, the fats will be part of your foods, as dressing for your vegetables, or as nuts and seeds sprinkled over your salad. And, as you know, oils run and spread all over the other foods.

But the Plate Method really does work. Try it a few times. Serve food onto your plate with a sense of how it should look according to this formula. In no time at all you will be using it—even at challenging eating situations, such as at a buffet, a potluck dinner, or at Grandma's house.

Thin-spiration _____

Use the Plate Method for teaching your children how to eat. Most likely, they'll relate better to the plate than the food pyramid. You can even have them make meal suggestions based on the Plate Method!

The Least You Need to Know

- The Traditional Food Pyramid currently in use is being updated by the government.

- The Food Guide Pyramid described in this chapter is designed for eating based on the glycemic index.

- Make most of your food selections from the lower two levels of the Food Guide Pyramid.

- Use the Plate Method for filling your plate at mealtimes and for teaching your children how to eat.

Chapter 8

Beginning Your Glycemic Index Weight-Loss Program

In This Chapter

◆ Choosing your best time

◆ Determining your goal size and weight

◆ Charting your progress

◆ Using a weight-loss journal

Now that you know the basics of glycemic index weight loss, you're probably excited about getting started. However, you might have some reservations about starting yet another diet program. By now, you may have been on enough diets to know that losing weight isn't exactly a cakewalk. You'll be making lifestyle changes, but you'll also be learning all about your body's biology in relation to carbohydrates and weight loss. This information will serve you well the rest of your life as you become one of those people who are naturally thin with a healthy and fit physique.

Can you do this? Of course you can! Thousands of people have been successful at not only losing weight, but also at keeping it off. As you know, the real success isn't losing the weight; it's staying at your ideal size for life.

Right this moment, tell yourself that you will be "healthy, happy, and the size I want to be." Then read on for some tips and tools to help you make that statement come true!

Timing Is Everything

In one sense, any time is the best time to lose weight. You don't want to wait one more second to make your excess weight disappear. Impatience can be an important advantage in weight loss. It means you're ready to do what it takes.

On the other hand, some times in life are better than others. You can set yourself up for success by reading through the following statements. If one or more are true for you, now may *not* be your best time to jump into a glycemic index weight-loss program:

◆ You need to lose weight quickly to look great at an upcoming event, such as a wedding or high school reunion. This kind of motivation often backfires, leading to yo-yo dieting, which never works. Think of glycemic index eating as a way of life, not as a means to quick weight loss.

◆ You don't have time in your life right now to give glycemic index weight loss the time and attention it requires.

◆ Your friend, spouse, doctor, or parent is urging you to lose weight. We applaud their suggestions to you, but unless you really want to lose weight, you aren't likely to succeed.

On the other hand, you're in great shape to get started if …

◆ You're starting a glycemic index weight-loss program of your own free will.

◆ You're committed to doing whatever it takes because you really want to live at your ideal size.

◆ You have the time and freedom to eat mostly low-glycemic foods.

◆ You want to go the distance, knowing that on any weight-loss program it can take months to lose weight and the rest of your life to keep it off.

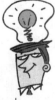

Thin-spiration

You can eat based on the glycemic index if you are pregnant or nursing, but you'll need a higher-glycemic load. Although eating mostly low-glycemic will benefit you and your baby, it is not recommended to start a weight-loss program during pregnancy or the first four months of nursing.

Good for you! You are in an ideal situation and state of mind to be successful, so let's get started.

Measurement Selection

You have many choices for measuring your progress. Although most people use weight scales to measure their progress, some are so turned off by the anxiety of stepping on the scales after many years of dieting that they prefer a different approach. We don't favor scales. Here is a variety of other measurement choices:

- **Monitor your measurements.** Before you start on your program, use a tape measure and record your chest or bust, waist, hips, upper thigh, and upper arm measurements. Then once a week or once every other week, take your measurements until you get to your ideal size. Then update them every month thereafter. If you want, set personal goals that outline what you want your ideal size and measurements to be.

- **Choose your ideal size.** If you're a man who felt great when he wore a size 36-inch belt, then set that as your goal. If you're a woman who yearns to be a size 8 again, set that as your goal. Find a pair of jeans that you would love to fit into. Try them on every week as you progress through the program. You'll know you've reached your goal right away when you can zip them up comfortably and also when you can sit down in them. Keep those jeans for life. Try them on every month or two to make sure you're staying at your ideal size.

- **Determine your ideal body fat percentage.** Lowering your body fat percentage is a healthful choice, so measuring it regularly is a good guide to overall health and fitness. You can have your body fat measured at a fitness center, health club, or health fair. There are many ways to measure body fat, such as with calipers, with a bio-impedance machine, and with underwater body measuring. All can meet your purpose, which is to measure the decrease in your body fat as you lose weight and tone up. The important thing is to have your body fat measured the same way every time. You'll get a more reliable measure of improvement.

Measure your body fat percentage at the start of your program and every two to three months thereafter.

Here's a chart that shows body fat percentages. Set your goal body fat percentage based on these ranges:

Status	Women	Men
Athlete level	17	10
Lean	17-22	10-15

Status	Women	Men
Normal	22-25	15-18
Above Normal	25-29	18-20
Overweight	29-35	20-25
Obese	over 35	over 25

The lower percentages are usually found in highly athletic individuals. If your body fat percentage is within the ideal range for your age, you don't need to be too concerned about your actual weight, because you'll look great and possess a higher metabolic rate.

◆ **Use the scale.** Weigh yourself once a week—no more—and preferably on the same day at the same time each week. Stepping on the scales daily isn't a good indicator of your progress because your weight can fluctuate too much from one day to the next and for seemingly no reason. Keep a notepad near the scales and record each week's weight. If you follow an exercise program, and we strongly advise you to get plenty of exercise, you'll be increasing your muscle mass. Muscle weighs more than fat, so your weight could be higher than you were expecting, but you'll be fitting comfortably into your clothes. This is actually a good situation because it means your basal metabolic rate is also higher. And the higher your metabolic rate, the easier it is for you to lose weight.

Thin-spiration _____

Most dieters who are hooked on "weighing in" every day don't take into account the fact that exercise will make you look better but may actually make you weigh more. That's because muscle weighs three times more than fat for the same amount of volume. So don't rely on the scale as the only measuring stick of success. You want to reduce your *size,* and converting bulky fat (which weighs less) into lean muscle (which weighs more) is the way to do it. The scale won't give you a true indication of your progress.

◆ **Calculate your body mass index (BMI).** This number is used by government agencies and health-care practitioners to determine whether a person is overweight and/or obese. If your BMI is between 25 and 29, you're considered to be overweight. If it's over 30, you're considered to be obese. You can use the chart that follows to determine your BMI.

BMI (kg/m²)	19	20	21	22	23	24	25	26	27	28	29	30	35	40
Height (in.)							Weight (lb.)							
58	91	96	100	105	110	115	119	124	129	134	138	143	167	191
59	94	99	104	109	114	119	124	128	133	138	143	148	173	198
60	97	102	107	112	118	123	128	133	138	143	148	153	179	204
61	100	106	111	116	122	127	132	137	143	148	153	158	185	211
62	104	109	115	120	126	131	136	142	147	153	158	164	191	218
63	107	113	118	124	130	135	141	146	152	158	163	169	197	225
64	110	116	122	128	134	140	145	151	157	163	169	174	204	232
65	114	120	126	132	138	144	150	156	162	168	174	180	210	240
66	118	124	130	136	142	148	155	161	167	173	179	186	216	247
67	121	127	134	140	146	153	159	166	172	178	185	191	223	255
68	125	131	138	144	151	158	164	171	177	184	190	197	230	262
69	128	135	142	149	155	162	169	176	182	189	196	203	236	270
70	132	139	146	153	160	167	174	181	188	195	202	207	243	278
71	136	143	150	157	165	172	179	186	193	200	208	215	250	286
72	140	147	154	162	169	177	184	191	199	206	213	221	258	294
73	144	151	159	166	174	182	189	197	204	212	219	227	265	302
74	148	155	163	171	179	186	194	202	210	218	225	233	272	311
75	152	160	168	176	184	192	200	208	216	224	232	240	279	319
76	156	164	172	180	189	197	205	213	221	230	238	246	287	328

The BMI is an excellent measurement, but it has some limitations. The formula penalizes someone who has lots of lean muscle. That's not good. If your body fat is low and your muscle mass is high, your BMI would put you into the overweight or obese category. In other words, highly muscled individuals who are definitely not overweight often have a high BMI because muscle weighs more. Most of us wish we had this problem! Any and all of these measurement gauges work. Which one you choose depends on what feels best to you. You can use all of them, one of them, or a combination. But by all means, measure your progress.

Setting Your Goal

The best way to set your weight or size goal is to be both realistic and optimistic. Realistic so that you can reach your goal, and optimistic to stay motivated. You never know what you can really achieve until you try your best!

If you are a woman who is 5'10" with a large frame, setting your goal as "I want to wear a size 6" is unrealistic. But perhaps a size 10 or 12 (maybe even size 8) is within the range of possibility. On the other hand, it would be a mistake for this woman to talk herself out of a size 10 or 12 and instead shoot for a size 16 if she really wants to recapture her youthful college-age silhouette. Her optimism to become a size 10 or 12 could actually propel her to reach her goal. You can always change your goal as you near your ideal size. And believe it or not, you do have a choice as to what size you'll be.

Be realistic about how long it will take for you to lose weight. This is *so* important! You already know your excess weight won't melt off overnight. In truth, it likely won't all come off in three months. Instead, plan on losing one or two pounds a week, or a dress or belt size every two months. You may progress faster or slower, so use these as estimates only. If this seems discouraging, just know that weight loss takes as long as it takes, but the end result—your ideal size—is yours to keep.

Thin-spiration

What's your hurry? Predictably, 9 times out of 10, yo-yo dieters are in a hurry to lose pounds, even lots of pounds. As Shakespeare would say, "That way lies madness." You didn't gain those 20 pounds in two months; don't try to lose them in two months. Although some people do successfully lose weight quickly, it's not the norm. Nor is it better. Slow, steady weight loss is more likely to last for the long term. And you won't be as tempted to quit just because you don't see huge reductions right away.

Set Up Your Journal

After you have determined how to track your progress, you need somewhere to track it. Purchase a journal or a spiral-bound notebook to use as your guidebook for your glycemic index weight loss. Depending on the amount of weight you want to lose and the length of time it takes, you might fill up several volumes.

Begin your journal by writing out your start date, your current size and weight, and your goals. Mark a section for recording your body's progress, another section to serve as a food diary, and a third section to track your exercise sessions.

Consider your journal to be very personal. After all, it's your history and it's also going to be filled with information that records your progress.

Thin-spiration

A journal is really, really valuable. Don't avoid creating one just because it seems like a hassle. Researchers have shown that people who record their food intake lose more weight than those who don't. You will learn a lot from your journal. By the way, don't "cheat" in your journal; it's just for you.

The Least You Need to Know

◆ Set a time to begin your glycemic index weight loss that fits into your schedule and personal needs.

◆ Choose your goal size and weight carefully, using pounds, how your jeans fit, body fat percentages, or BMI.

◆ Usc a daily food diary to record your food intake and to keep you on track.

Chapter 9

Get Your Mind Aligned

In This Chapter

- ◆ Harnessing your mental powers
- ◆ Writing weight-loss affirmations
- ◆ Banishing past weight-loss failures
- ◆ Connecting with new eating behaviors

Attempting any weight-loss program can be either inspiring or depressing. The difference depends on you and your attitude. Based on all the scientific research, glycemic index weight loss is extraordinarily effective and safe. Yet even on a low-glycemic plan, some people succeed at losing weight and maintaining their ideal size for life, and some people don't.

You want to be one of those who succeed. You want to be someone who lives a healthy life at your ideal size. So it's important to use all the tools available, including the power of your mind.

In this chapter, you learn how to actively employ your innate mental power throughout your entire weight-loss and maintenance experience. It's readily available, it's totally free, and it will do exactly what you want it to do. All you need is to tell your mind what to think.

Your Private Weight-Loss Ally

Many diet programs, this book included, tell you exactly what and when to eat to lose weight. Most teach you all you need to know about how your biology works to gain, store, and lose fat. But you need more. Your ultimate success depends on one factor of your biology seldom mentioned in any dieting or weight-loss program—your mind.

Your mind is your innate mental power. The power of your mind is far greater than your willpower and self-discipline. In fact, right now your willpower and self-discipline are likely strong enough for you to start on a low-glycemic weight-loss program.

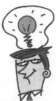

Thin-spiration

Time and again, we hear of athletes who first visualize their competitive goals, then talk positively about their goals, and ultimately reach their goals. The same can be true for you in your weight-loss efforts.

But you need to follow up your determination with positive thinking and a positive mental attitude. Positive thinking isn't simply a good idea for motivation, it's a necessity. Self-talk is actually a self-fulfilling prophecy. What you think you'll achieve is exactly what you will achieve. But first you need to take an honest look at your inner thoughts about your weight and your weight-loss history.

The Ghost of Weight-Loss Past

Whether you call them ghosts or skeletons, after years of dealing with weight issues, you are haunted by past failures. Unfortunately, they can seem to predict your future, and that prediction can be anything but positive, uplifting, and inspiring. In fact, it can be bleak. The first step in using your mental power to reach your goals is to identify your negative self-talk.

You might already doubt yourself with such questions and statements as …

- ◆ What makes me think I can succeed this time?
- ◆ How can I possibly deprive myself of all my favorite junk foods? Not just for now, but forever?
- ◆ I have fat genes.
- ◆ Everyone in my family is fat.
- ◆ I have no willpower.

◆ I might lose my friends if I lose weight.

◆ It's too expensive to eat low-glycemic foods.

◆ I've lost and gained the same 50 pounds over and over again.

◆ I hate vegetables.

◆ As I get older, I'm just naturally getting bigger.

◆ I was overweight as a child, so I don't know what it would be like not to be fat.

You get the dialogue. It goes on and on, and you can probably think of many more statements or questions to add to the previous list. In a sense, all negative self-talk has an element of truth to it. But negative self-talk is also deceptive, because these thoughts are the very thoughts that have held you and your body back from living at your ideal size. They've literally made themselves true.

After identifying the negative self-talk about your size, weight, and eating, the next step is to convert those statements into what you want to be true.

> **CAUTION**
>
> **Wrong Weigh**
>
> Avoid the very real temptation to feel guilty and blame yourself if you don't stick to your glycemic index weight-loss eating plans. Losing weight is at best an imperfect process. If you overeat or eat incorrectly, forgive yourself so that you banish guilt and discouragement. Instead, refocus your energy and eat according to plan at your next meal.

Creating New Thoughts

For every negative statement of self-talk, there is an opposite, positive statement. Your mission is to turn around your thoughts so that you actually affirm what you want.

For example, the opposite positive of "I hate vegetables" is "I love vegetables." Now, now, instead of saying "Oh, yuck" to yourself, think again. If you continue to hate vegetables, this low-glycemic weight-loss program is going to be painful, unpleasant, and short-lived. If you essentially convince yourself that you love vegetables, however, you're going to love eating the low-glycemic way.

Although it might seem untrue, you can change virtually any thought you have, and only you can do it. The same goes for losing weight. No one else can do it for you.

The same can be true for any thought. Take the statement "It's too expensive to eat low-glycemic foods." Turn it around to "Eating low-glycemic foods fits well within my food budget." Only then will you discover that it can actually cost less to eat low-glycemic foods—such as a side salad at a fast-food drive-through rather than a pricier burger, fries, and soda.

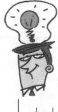

Thin-spiration

If you tell yourself that you love vegetables, your subconscious will come to believe this. You're going to find yourself requesting a double order of broccoli or zucchini at restaurants. And, of all wonders, they'll be satisfying and delicious.

The main benefit to rewriting the negative statements into positive ones is that you gain the power and momentum to reach your goals. And you'll eventually do it with more ease, less frustration, and more confidence.

In the beginning pages of your weight-loss journal, write down your biggest objections and self-doubts. Then underneath each one write the opposite positive. Review the list whenever you feel discouraged or want to toss out the cabbage or green beans and head to the neighborhood bakery for éclairs and crème puffs.

Your Personal Affirmations

As you begin to make the necessary mental shifts in self-talk, you need a concise set of personal affirmations. Affirmations are forward-thinking statements written in the present tense.

You can choose from the following or make up a set of your own:

♦ I enjoy living and eating the low-glycemic way.

♦ I am now at my ideal size and I will easily stay at my ideal size for life. (Use this affirmation even if you aren't already at your ideal size. You are actually programming your subconscious to do the inner work to get you there.)

♦ I am now enjoying the health benefits of eating the low-glycemic way.

♦ I am comfortable and safe at my ideal size.

♦ I am successful and happy at my ideal size.

♦ I love, honor, and appreciate my body.

♦ I enjoy exercise.

- ◆ I exercise vigorously three to four times a week.

- ◆ I enjoy eating and preparing low-glycemic meals and snacks.

- ◆ I am in harmony with being at my ideal size.

- ◆ I easily eat low-glycemic meals when dining out, on vacations, and when traveling.

- ◆ My body feels great when I eat low-glycemic foods.

And try this one on for size:

I have skinny genes. Or is it skinny jeans? Of course, it's both!

Affirmations are powerful tools. On a low-glycemic eating program, affirmations are as essential as meats and vegetables.

But affirmations are only powerful if you use them. After you have a complete list, you need to start using them on a daily basis. Remember, it doesn't matter whether your list seems within the realm of possibility. In fact, it probably shouldn't be. Quite honestly, your affirmations should sound far-fetched and outrageous. If you were already living them, you would probably already be at your ideal size.

> **Body of Knowledge**
>
> You can use affirmations for other aspects of your life. Use them for success with your work, relationships, and health. Just be sure that your affirmations are positive, present tense, and that they preferably start with "I am."

Keep your list with you. Write affirmations in your journal, post them on your computer, and key them into your PDA. Post them in the kitchen and on your desk at work. And if your car often serves as a kitchen table away from home, post them on the dashboard.

At least once a day, and preferably twice, say each affirmation out loud. Set aside your incredulity and just say them. You'll soon get in the flow of their power, and eating the low-glycemic way will become second nature to you. Your results will prove your former inner-self doubts wrong.

A Treasure Map

Living at your ideal size has probably been a goal of yours for a long time. Attainment is within your grasp. Setting up visual cues supports your goal. Do this by creating a "treasure map." It can be as elaborate or as simple as you like.

A simple treasure map might contain just one image—a picture that represents you at your ideal size. It might be a picture of you in earlier days when you were at your ideal size. It can also be a picture of a thin man or woman cut out from a magazine, perhaps with your face superimposed on the image.

Your treasure map can consist of one or more images in different locations, or you can create an elaborate, poster-sized treasure map with pictures of yourself, your favorite low-glycemic foods, and even pictures of a dream beach vacation you want to take.

Thin-spiration

As you put together your treasure map, remember that you're in this for the long run. Add pictures of what you'll be doing next year, and the year after that, and also add pictures of the low-glycemic foods that you enjoy the most.

Paste a motivating picture or pictures in your journal. You might also want to paste in a "before" photo and "progress" photos. Paste a motivational picture wherever you'll see it frequently. The bathroom mirror is a good place, and you can use the picture as a desktop image on your computer.

A treasure map keeps you focused on your goal and makes living through the details of getting there a whole lot easier.

Real-Time Concerns

Even though low-glycemic weight loss is a terrific choice for weight loss, a time might come when you doubt yourself and your program. Don't let doubts and discouragements prevent you from attaining your ideal size. Instead, use them as a springboard.

First, recognize that the part of you that's speaking at the moment is the Ghost of Weight-Loss Past. This scary ghost comes from your mischievous brain remembering past emotions and frustrations—which is really what it's programmed to do. So it's okay to acknowledge what that old ghost has to say, but it's not okay to take action just yet.

Instead, ignore that ghost for a moment and ask yourself—your current powerful, committed, and enthusiastic self—what you want. The answer is to attain your ideal size and to go the distance. Your powerful self can turn around the situation right then and there by saying aloud your list of affirmations.

This is exactly why you need to keep your affirmations close at hand all the time, because you never know when that ghost is going to appear.

Modeling "Thin" Behaviors

You didn't become overweight by eating like a thin person. No one does. Right now, social scientists who study weight issues and obesity are turning their attention to the 35 percent of the U.S. population who are naturally at their ideal size. To give others a model to go by, these researchers are looking for the behavior patterns of people who have been successful in controlling their weight.

Here's a list of "thin" behaviors to model:

♦ Eat when your body is truly hungry and avoid eating when prompted by television advertising, donut day at the office, or other feeding opportunities. After a few times of saying "no," it becomes remarkably easier.

♦ Sit down when you eat. Rather than stand at the kitchen counter or over the stove, pull up a seat and relax enough to enjoy your food.

♦ Rather than snack mindlessly when you're watching television or working on your computer, keep food in the kitchen and away from entertainment centers.

♦ Completely clear out high-glycemic snacks from your desk at work (veggie snacks can substitute), and never eat in your car.

♦ Develop an aversion to overeating and that stuffed feeling in your stomach.

♦ When you go out to eat, split an entrée with your spouse, children, or whomever you are with. No one needs that much food. And, of course, you can split a dessert four or five ways. You'll find that a bite or two can be just as satisfying, and perhaps even more satisfying, than the whole piece of cheesecake.

♦ When dining alone, ask for a half-serving, or only eat half—or less—and take the remaining food home. (You can also ask for a take-home box at the start of the meal and immediately put half away. Out of sight, out of mind, and best of all, the food's not in your mouth.)

♦ Eat slowly. Don't rush. Savor your food.

♦ Avoid making eating your entertainment or your therapist. Instead, develop healthier outlets for fun and comfort.

♦ Become a picky eater and never make a point of cleaning your plate. Eat what you need to eat.

As you adopt these behaviors, you'll find that it's easier to go the distance with low-glycemic weight loss and you'll have fewer moments of missing "the good old overeating days."

The Least You Need to Know

♦ Your mental power is a terrific asset for losing weight and keeping it off.

♦ Use affirmations to harness the power of your mind and to stay on track with your low-glycemic weight-loss program.

♦ Chart your weight-loss progress by using posters and graphs.

♦ Model the behaviors of thin people to jump-start your program.

10

Your Glycemic Index Weight-Loss Program

In This Chapter

♦ Discovering the Keep It Simple program

♦ Learning the Comprehensive program

♦ Making adjustments

♦ Maintaining your weight

There's no time like the present. That is especially true when embarking on a new eating plan based on the glycemic index.

If you've read this far, you're ready. You understand the basics of the glycemic index. You've learned some fundamental aspects of weight loss. And you're determined to successfully lose weight and keep it off.

In this chapter, we give you two methods for using the glycemic index to lose weight. The first program is simple and easy because you don't need to count or calculate; however, your food choices are more limited. The second program is more detailed, but it offers you more food choices. You decide which one works best for you.

Be sure that you choose one or the other of these glycemic index programs. Don't mix the two because you could have negative results. You can certainly switch programs anytime you like, but then stick with that program for at least four weeks before you make another change.

Both choices give you room to savor and enjoy delicious foods while you keep your fat-burning mechanism revved up, allowing you to lose weight safely and easily.

Two Glycemic Eating Programs

Forget what you've heard about *induction phases*, or three-phase weight-loss programs. With glycemic index weight loss, there is only one phase. This means that you'll use the same program to initially lose weight and to continue your weight loss. You may need to adjust the program as you move into lifelong weight maintenance, but you can stick with the same basic program.

Glyco Lingo

An **induction phase** is a standard part of low-carb weight-loss programs. In the two-week induction phase, a person eats strictly limited amounts of carbohydrates, most of which are "free vegetables." Induction phase eating is out of balance and not necessary for weight loss.

Eating based on the glycemic index can be intricate and complex or it can be simple. If you don't have time in your life to count, weigh, and measure, use the first program—Keep It Simple. If you prefer a more rigorous program, use the second program—Comprehensive. Either way, you'll be able to reach your weight-loss goals.

Program One—Keep It Simple

The first program will work best for you if you have always wanted a weight-loss program that's stunningly simple. Here are some other ways to know if you want simple and easy:

◆ You don't have time to keep a detailed food diary.

◆ You are very busy or live a high-stress life.

◆ You frequently eat at restaurants, travel, or lead a hectic social life.

◆ You are allergic to or have food sensitivities to wheat or gluten or you have *celiac disease*. Although these aren't common health conditions, if you need to avoid wheat or gluten and need to lose weight, the Keep It Simple program will work for you.

◆ You cook for a full family—spouse, children, and others.

If "keeping it simple" is how you wish you could live, then use this program.

Glyco Lingo

Celiac disease is a chronic digestive disorder that's caused by intolerance to gluten. Gluten is found in wheat, spelt, rye, oats, and barley. Most common in Caucasians of European descent, people with celiac disease need to avoid eating foods that contain gluten, because it can be life-threatening.

What to Eat

The food and eating guidelines for the Keep It Simple program give you plenty of choices. You definitely won't feel starved, but you also need to eat modest quantities if you want those pounds to come off. Here's what to eat.

◆ For each meal, eat about three to four ounces of animal protein and two to three servings of vegetables. You can substitute one fruit for one vegetable. The protein fills about $1/4$ of your plate.

◆ Make your vegetable servings fill about half your plate at each meal. Yes, that means trying to eat plenty of vegetables, even for breakfast.

◆ The remaining part of your plate, or about $1/4$, can contain low-glycemic fruit, low-glycemic dairy products, such as milk or yogurt, or low-glycemic starches, such as yams, legumes, sweet potatoes, and winter squash. Obviously, you wouldn't pour milk on your plate, but the milk could be about $1/4$ of your meal.

Body of Knowledge

Three to four ounces of meat, seafood, or poultry contains about 18 to 28 grams of protein. Three ounces is about the size of a deck of cards or the size of a small can of tuna. That's all the protein an average-size woman—the size you may want to be if you're a woman—needs to eat three times a day to stay healthy. It's best not to eat much more than that. An average-size man can eat four ounces of protein three times a day. In other words, forget about ordering the 16-ounce ribeye at the steak house ... unless you plan to feed four or five people!

◆ Select one small serving of a treat food per day. The treat food can be high-glycemic, but you'll lose weight faster if it's low-glycemic. Eat a serving a day. Treat foods are such goodies as ice cream, custard, cheesecake, a candy bar, or chocolate. The lower your treat is on the glycemic index, the better. Yes, you can spread out your treat over the course of a day, but limit yourself to a total of only one serving. Unfortunately, you can't define a serving of premium ice cream as the entire carton—it's ½ cup.

◆ Fat fills about 10 percent of your plate but in reality, most of it's already part of the other foods you're eating, such as butter on your cooked vegetables and the natural fat found in meats and fish.

◆ Avoid eating all high-glycemic and medium-glycemic starches including white potatoes, white breads, some rice, and all refined products made with wheat. For starches, you can eat legumes, sweet potatoes, yams, and winter squash. And you can eat modest amounts of thick-cut oats, 100 percent bran, and corn and corn products each week—but alas, not popcorn, unless you choose it as one of your treat foods for the week (but watching the amount will be important). Later on, you can add back some starches—more on that in the maintenance section of this chapter.

Wrong Weigh _____

If you can't eat just one small serving of a treat food per day without wanting to overeat, then don't eat the treat food. Most of the time when a person starts eating based on the glycemic index they learn to enjoy just a couple bites of a treat food. If your treat foods are also trigger foods, stay away from them until you feel more confident about controlling the amount you eat.

Thin-spiration _____

Luscious dark chocolate has a glycemic index value of 48, which is low-glycemic. It can make an ideal treat if you love chocolate and keep your serving size to two ounces.

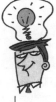

Thin-spiration _____

Yes, you can live well and healthy and even happily without eating starches, or by eating very few. On the Keep It Simple program, you need to eat starches selectively and with discretion. If you have a favorite starch food, such as donuts or chocolate cake, you can have a normal-size piece of your treat food occasionally. Be sure you don't waste your treat food on a starch you don't really love. In other words, don't eat that tempting slice of breakfast toast, unless you really love toast.

CAUTION

Wrong Weigh

Popcorn, unlike most corn products, is high-glycemic at 72. For most of us, the challenge is the serving size. A serving of 1½ cups of popcorn has a glycemic load of 8. But who ever eats that little? Even a medium popcorn purchased at the movies would contain 5 or 6 cups. Other corn products, such as fresh or frozen corn and corn chips, have a low- to medium-glycemic index. You can eat a couple servings of them each week. Corn, like the other carbohydrate foods, will fit that ¼ of the plate intended for higher-glycemic foods.

◆ Eat low-glycemic snacks such as nuts, nut butters, dried fruit, olives, dill pickles, meats, and cheeses. Also enjoy hard-boiled eggs, deviled eggs, or pickled eggs, or try raw vegetables with cheese dip. Read through the list of low-glycemic foods and nonstarchy veggies and select the ones you enjoy most.

On the Keep It Simple program, eat small amounts of whole-fat salad dressings, butter, olive oil, spices, seasonings, and condiments. Spices, seasonings, and most condiments are "free foods." The serving size for the fats is one teaspoon oil or butter, and one tablespoon for salad dressing, 6 to 10 nuts, one tablespoon of seeds, and ¼ small avocado. Eat no more than six servings of fats per day. For beverages, drink purified water and herbal teas. You can consume one cup of caffeinated beverages such as tea and coffee if you choose. Late afternoon lattes could count as your one cup of caffeine—order them up with whole milk or skim milk.

Fine Tuning

As you begin to eat on the Keep It Simple program, only check your body size or your weight once every week. If you haven't seen a difference after two weeks, you may need to make one or more of the following adjustments:

◆ Cut out corn products. Especially if the corn products you're eating are medium-glycemic instead of low. If you are eating corn chips, they generally contain added fats and thus added calories and may be the culprit.

◆ Take a hard look at your quantities and lower your serving sizes, especially of the higher-carbohydrate foods. These include fruit, milk, yogurt, grain foods, and starchy vegetables.

◆ Choose a low- to medium–glycemic treat instead of one that's high-glycemic.

◆ Reduce your stress levels. See Chapter 23.

If these changes don't work, start keeping a detailed food diary and you will probably figure out what's not working. It's easy to get a bit sloppy when you don't keep notes. But one of the beauties of the Keep It Simple program is that you don't need to keep notes.

Foods to Eat Sparingly

As you eat the Keep It Simple way, here's a list of foods to avoid or eat very infrequently:

◆ High-glycemic foods.

◆ Fruit juices. Eat fruit instead. The fiber in the fruit slows digestion so the glycemic index and load are lower. If you want juice, you can mix juice with water in the ratio of about $^1/_3$ juice to $^2/_3$ water and have one glass two or three times a week, preferably with a meal.

◆ Aspartame and other artificial sweeteners. Some research shows they stimulate appetite. Other research indicates they aren't health-promoting. Aspartame is in diet sodas and many other diet products. It's also used as a sweetener in yogurt and processed puddings and custards.

◆ Coffee and caffeine. If you love your morning coffee or tea, eat breakfast while you savor your "wake-up" brew.

◆ Alcoholic beverages. Limit yourself to one to two drinks a week. Alcoholic beverages can stimulate appetite so they could derail your weight-loss efforts. But not everyone reacts the same way.

◆ Soft drinks and sodas. Instead drink water or herbal teas. If you crave flavor in your water, add a slice of lemon, lime, or orange.

◆ Any food that you're allergic to or sensitive to.

Eating these foods can stall your weight loss or lead to weight-loss plateaus. If you reach a plateau, make sure that you aren't eating these foods and start keeping a food and beverage journal for a couple days. Most likely, you'll figure out what you're doing wrong.

The Comprehensive Program

The Comprehensive glycemic index weight-loss program incorporates all the details and nuances of the glycemic index. Choose the Comprehensive program if you …

◆ Want to or need to keep detailed eating records.

◆ Have an analytical mind and value precision.

◆ Have the time and energy to add up your food intake based on glycemic load.

◆ Are willing to make modifications to the program based on your rate of weight loss.

◆ Need structure. Research shows that people who keep track of more detail and write down their food intake during their weight-loss program do better.

> **Thin-spiration**
>
> To determine the glycemic load of your foods, you don't need a sharp pencil and calculator, but rather a good glycemic index list. The lists now include the glycemic load for average serving sizes. You can use the list in Appendix B at the back of this book.

How Much to Eat

In the Comprehensive program, you'll be keeping track of your glycemic load. To start, you need to keep track of your food intake. Use this chart.

Time	Food or Beverage	Amount	Glycemic Index	Glycemic Load	Total by Meal

Totals by Day _____   **Glycemic Load Units** _____

Your goal is to eat 60 to 75 glycemic load units a day. You'll be eating about 15 to 20 each for breakfast, lunch, and dinner. An extra 15 to 20 are for snacks during the day. You can have two or three snacks per day.

You'll need a notebook to keep your daily tally sheets. Plus, you'll need a good and reliable glycemic index, glycemic load chart, and carbohydrate gram chart. You can download the glycemic index with glycemic load from www.mendosa.com. The site has computer software you can order, too. With GlycoLoad, from www.phelpsteam. com/glycoload, your computer automatically calculates the glycemic load of any amount of food as long as you know how many ounces you plan to eat. You can also use the glycemic index and glycemic load listing in Appendix B of this book. And, you can use the list in the book *What Makes My Blood Glucose Go Up … and Down* by Jennie Brand-Miller.

> **Body of Knowledge**
>
> If you choose to count carbohy-drate grams, you can have between 90 to 150 grams of carbohydrates a day. Choose all or at least 85 percent of your foods from the low-glycemic index list only. You'll be having 30 grams of carbohydrates for breakfast, lunch, and dinner, and be using between 10 to 30 grams of carbohydrates for two to three snacks a day.

> **Wrong Weigh**
>
> Don't save up glycemic load units or carbohydrate grams and then eat them all at one meal. This defeats the purpose of glycemic index weight loss. If you do this, you'll send your blood sugar and insulin levels soaring and your body will be inclined to respond by storing fat rather than by releasing it.

What to Eat

On the Comprehensive program, you'll limit high-glycemic carbohydrates to less than 15 percent of your carbohydrate intake every day. Eat mostly low-glycemic carbohydrates or "free foods" and perhaps some medium-glycemic foods.

Your meals will look like this:

- At each meal, fill half of your plate with non-starchy vegetables. For breakfast, you can substitute one fruit for a vegetable provided that the glycemic load for each meal is 25 or less.

- Eat about three to four ounces of animal protein. This is about the size of a deck of cards or a small can of tuna. Choose from meats, seafood, poultry, and eggs. Men can eat four ounces.

- You can eat breads, crackers, and pastas made with stone-ground or coarse-ground grains, and so on; just be sure that they're low-glycemic. Cook pasta al dente, about 5 to 6 minutes and no longer. When you can, eat genuine stone-ground breads. Ditto that for crackers and muffins.

◆ Include dairy products, such as milk, yogurt, and cheese, keeping within your daily glycemic load recommendations. Plain yogurt and milk contain between 12 to 17 grams of carbohydrates per serving and have glycemic loads of about 2 to 4. One serving is one cup. Cheese has a 0 glycemic load and is mainly protein, so use it as part of your total protein food allotment. Eat no more than 1 ounce of cheese a day, or less.

Thin-spiration

When computing the glycemic load of a meal, you can reduce the count by one third if you eat at least four teaspoons of vinegar in your salad dressing. That means your glycemic load per meal could be as high as 37 if you go ahead and eat that tangy salad.

◆ Dessert can be a low-glycemic food, such as premium ice cream or fruit. Remember, though, to keep your food intake within 15 to 20 glycemic load units for each meal if you're eating a total of 60 to 75 glycemic load units per day.

Snacks can include stone-ground whole grain crackers with cheese, dried fruit, and vegetables and fruit. You can also choose snacks from the nonstarchy veggies list.

Monitoring Your Progress

On the Comprehensive glycemic index weight-loss program, you may need to adjust your total glycemic load for the day. If you find that, after eating 60 to 75 glycemic load units a day for two weeks or so, you aren't losing weight, then you'll need to lower your glycemic load units. If you are counting carbohydrate grams instead of glycemic load units, you can lower your carb grams to as little as 15 per meal instead of 30 per meal.

Thin-spiration

If you want to accelerate your weight loss, increase the amount of fiber you eat up to 30 grams per day. You can also add more acidic foods to your meals, as a way to lower the effective glycemic load.

You can lower the glycemic load unit amount to 50 or even 40, but we don't recommend going lower than 40 per day. Continue to balance the load throughout the day. So if you choose to eat 50 units, then divide them as follows: 10 to 15 for each meal and 5 to 15 for snacks.

Weight-Loss Expectations

Basically, there's no way to predict how fast you'll lose weight. Some factors that could make a difference are …

- ◆ **Age.** A general rule of thumb is that it takes longer to lose weight when a person is older because one's metabolism slows with age.

- ◆ **Current weight.** If you have lots of weight to lose, your initial weight loss could be faster than a person who only has 15 to 20 pounds to lose.

- ◆ **Metabolic rate.** If your body fat percentage is high, it could take longer than if it's low. If you have been told that you're metabolically resistant to weight loss, increase your strength-training exercise to lower body fat percentage and boost metabolism.

- ◆ **Food sensitivities and allergies.** Avoid eating these foods to speed up your weight loss.

Body of Knowledge

If you suspect that you have food allergies or food sensitivities, here's what you can do. Set an appointment with an allergist to test for possible food allergies. You can also avoid eating that food for a week and if your symptoms are gone, then try to cut that food out of your diet. But if you suspect that you are sensitive to more than one food, consulting with an allergist can help you unravel your body's reactions.

If you want to speed up your weight loss, be sure to read through this book and follow the suggestions to boost your metabolism, reduce stress, and use the power of your mind.

Don't be afraid of losing weight too fast with glycemic index weight loss. The meals you're eating are balanced, nutritious, and wholesome, so there's no danger that you'll be starving yourself.

Maintaining Your Weight Loss

The good news is that you can easily maintain your weight loss by continuing to eat based on the glycemic index. You'll keep doing what you're doing right now, but your food intake will be more liberal.

◆ On the Keep It Simple maintenance program, you can add one serving of low-glycemic grain-based food such as bread, rice, or pasta, if you don't have celiac disease or allergies to gluten or wheat. Try this for two weeks. If you continue to lose weight, add one more serving of dairy or a low-glycemic grain.

◆ On the Comprehensive maintenance program, you'll increase your glycemic load units by 20 for two weeks. If you're still losing weight, increase by 20 until you have stopped losing weight. Continue to balance the glycemic load among all three meals and snacks.

Keep your food portions the same for meats, seafood, and poultry—about three to four ounces per meal. You'll never need to eat more than this amount. Continue to fill half your plate at each meal with nonstarchy vegetables.

The Least You Need to Know

◆ You can choose between the Keep It Simple or the Comprehensive programs for glycemic index weight loss.

◆ Fill half your plate with nonstarchy vegetables at each meal.

◆ Eat mostly low-glycemic carbohydrates and only rarely eat high-glycemic carbs.

◆ The maintenance programs are a relaxed version of the program you have chosen.

Part 3

Nutritionally Balanced Eating

Your meal-planning emphasis is now centered around eating moderate amounts of meats, seafood, poultry, and eggs along with 5 to 10 servings of vegetables and fruits every day plus stone-ground breads, whole grains, and low-glycemic cereals. Make wise choices for animal protein and good fats. Learn how to incorporate dairy into your meals and find ways to enjoy sweet tastes without reverting to white sugars, white flours, and junk foods. Supplement your food intake with nutritional and dietary supplements that give you support for glycemic index weight loss. Investigate supplements that enhance your digestion, plus those that soothe moods and balance your electrolytes.

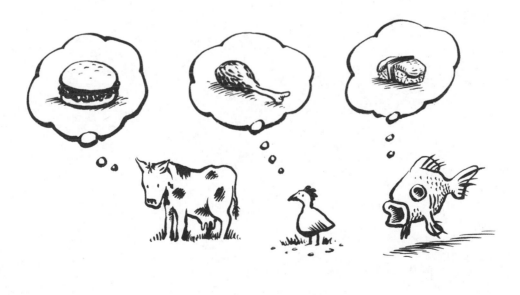

Protein

In This Chapter

- Understanding the importance of proteins
- Using proper serving sizes
- Eating as a vegetarian
- Stocking your pantry

Perhaps you've been on one of those popular diet programs that urges you to eat as much meat and fat as you desire. Breakfast could have been $^1/_2$ pound of fried bacon and four or even six eggs, and the results were promising—you could lose some weight. But you weren't eating healthily. In fact, you could have been doing your body as much harm as good.

Things have definitely changed in the world of weight loss. You don't need to rush out to the grocery store to purchase massively huge sirloin steaks, rashers of bacon, and mountains of ground beef to lose weight. Instead, dine on moderate amounts of succulent meats, seafood, poultry, and eggs.

In this chapter, you learn how much protein and which kinds of protein your body requires to lose weight and maintain good health plus a high metabolism.

Your Body Needs Protein

When a person is accustomed to eating high-carbohydrate and high-glycemic foods, protein becomes an afterthought. You might center your meals around pastas, breads, or potatoes. Or, like many of us, around what we thought was the only reason for eating a meal—the dessert.

What a mistake! Meals aren't supposed to be about indulging a sweet (or starch) tooth, but about eating important nutrients that support your health and well-being. We know now that one of the reasons people become overweight is because they missed the point.

The point is that each meal needs to include high-quality *complete protein*. Your body needs protein daily, and preferably three times a day. That's how you receive the all-important essential *amino acids* that are the building blocks of your body. They build muscle. They boost metabolism. They keep your hair, skin, and fingernails lustrous and glowing. And here's more:

Glyco Lingo

Complete protein is protein that contains adequate amounts of all nine essential amino acids. Only animal proteins, such as meats, seafood, eggs, and dairy, can provide this.

Glyco Lingo

Amino acids are the chemical units that form proteins. They make up the muscles, ligaments, tendons, organs, glands, nails, hair, and even vital body fluids. They also help regulate all bodily and metabolic processes. The body needs to obtain nine essential amino acids through food regularly for good health.

- Proteins make up muscles, ligaments, tendons, organs, glands, nails, and hair, and are essential for strong bones.

- Proteins help regulate the body's water balance and maintain the proper internal pH balance. A lack of protein can cause water retention and edema.

- Proteins form the structural basis of DNA.

- Without adequate protein, the strength of your immune system is jeopardized.

- Proteins in the form of amino acids activate vitamin and mineral utilization by the body.

- Eating the right amount of protein assists your body in losing weight and maintaining weight loss.

- Proteins rebuild and restore body tissue and muscle.

◆ Eating protein slows down the digestion of sugars and starches and helps prevent a rapid rise in blood sugar levels.

As you can see from the previous list, you don't want to skimp on eating proteins. Instead, make sure that you eat some animal protein at every meal.

The Nine Essential Amino Acids

Only by eating high-quality protein can you obtain the nine essential amino acids found in food that are essential to bodily functions. The other 20 or so amino acids your body needs are manufactured in the liver by using the nine essential amino acids as the raw materials. Without the essential nine, your body simply won't perform properly.

> **Body of Knowledge**
>
> Eating protein is vital to the liver's health and function. Fasting has been promoted as a way to lose weight and detoxify the body, but not eating enough protein actually prevents the liver from detoxifying. Fasting has never been shown to be a healthful or effective means for long-term weight loss.

Types of Animal Proteins

For your glycemic index weight-loss program, eat animal protein at least three times a day. You can savor the following animal proteins:

◆ **Meats.** Beef, pork, buffalo, lamb, veal, and wild game such as venison, moose, and elk.

◆ **Poultry.** Chicken, turkey, duck, Cornish game hens, along with wild game such as pheasant, quail, geese, duck, and doves.

◆ **Seafood.** Shellfish such as crab, shrimp, lobster, calamari, mussels, and clams, plus all fish found in oceans, streams, and lakes. This includes salmon, sardines, trout, bass, tuna, snapper, and the list goes on and on.

◆ **Eggs.** Eat the entire egg; both yolk and white contain protein.

◆ **Dairy.** The only dairy product that contains virtually no carbohydrates is regular hard cheese, such as cheddar, Edam, feta, and Swiss. Cottage cheese and feta

 Wrong Weigh

Because some egg substitutes contain additives, you may want to avoid any form of eggs that come as liquid. Go totally natural and crack your own when you can.

cheese contain about 6 grams of carbohydrates per cup. Low-fat cheeses, including low-fat cottage cheese, contain about 8 grams of carbohydrates per cup. Unsweetened dairy products have a low-glycemic index. Milk and yogurt offer you some protein, but not as much as other animal protein sources. Don't use milk or yogurt as your primary source of protein for a meal.

Vegetable Proteins

You might already know that soy products contain protein, as do many other vegetables. All legumes and nuts contain a significant amount of protein, and soybeans are legumes. But when you're eating the glycemic index way, vegetable protein also counts as carbohydrates. The glycemic index of vegetable proteins, such as legumes, is low—usually ranging between 14 to 25.

Vegetable proteins are not complete proteins; they're *incomplete proteins*. They don't give your body everything it needs in the realm of protein, and often the protein in the food is difficult for humans to digest and assimilate.

Glyco Lingo

Incomplete proteins are foods that don't contain all nine essential amino acids in optimal quantities. These foods are vegetables or vegetable-based, such as soybeans, nuts, legumes, and grains.

Vegetarians often use food combining as a way to obtain adequate amounts of essential amino acids from vegetables. They combine a legume with a grain into a dish, such as red beans and rice.

Food combining doesn't work well for eating based on the glycemic index. By the time a person finishes eating enough "brown rice and beans" to provide 20 grams of complete protein, the glycemic load would be off the acceptable chart for that meal.

Wrong Weigh

Soy products offer you essential amino acids, but not at optimal levels. Soy is limited in methionine and tryptophan. Health-wise, small amounts of soy might be okay, but large consumption of soy products has been linked to thyroid malfunction and dementia. Soy products, such as roasted soybeans and tempeh are fine for your maintenance program, but should be counted as carbohydrates and not protein. We recommend eating only one to four servings per week. You'll learn more about soy in Chapter 14.

Serving Sizes

Your body's need for complete protein depends on the size of your frame and your activity level. Don't worry, there's no need for challenging calculations here. We make it simple.

Men need about 4 to 5 ounces of animal protein three times a day. Women need about 3 to 4 ounces. For women, that's an amount equal to the size of a deck of cards or a small can of tuna. Men need as much animal protein as 1½ decks of cards.

If a person orders a 16-ounce rib-eye steak for dinner, that's enough protein to feed four adults.

> **CAUTION**
>
> **Wrong Weigh**
>
> If you want to substitute cottage cheese for meat and fish, use these guidelines. An ounce of meat or fish is equivalent in protein to ¼ cup cottage cheese.

You don't need to eat more than the recommended amount. In fact, it's best if you don't overdo it. Overeating anything causes increased insulin levels, and it's now been found that eating too much protein over a long period of time can lead to insulin resistance. Some animal proteins also contain a significant amount of fat, and too much fat causes more insulin resistance. When a person is insulin-resistant, weight loss becomes more difficult.

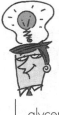

> **Thin-spiration**
>
> It's a common misconception that eating the low-glycemic way is more expensive than eating a high-carbohydrate and high-glycemic all-purpose diet. But if you sharpen your pencil and calculate the difference between eggs and fruit versus cereal, milk, and juice for breakfast, the costs are just about equal. And if you include all the money spent on junk foods, sodas, and candy machines, low-glycemic eating may cost you less.

When you eat protein, the body releases small amounts of insulin, but not nearly the same amount as when you eat carbohydrates. When people eat excessive amounts of animal protein, however, not only do they increase their fat intake, but their insulin can rise far enough to affect fat storage. As you are learning, making sure you eat the right amount of each type of food is important for ultimate weight-loss success.

Vegetarian Choices

Being a vegan—a person who eats no animal proteins—and eating for a glycemic index and a desirable glycemic load weight-loss program are fundamentally incompatible. Eating mostly only vegetables and grains or grain-based products won't result in the weight loss you desire. However, people who embrace a modified vegetarian philosophy can be quite successful eating the low-glycemic way, especially if they eat fish, poultry, eggs, and cheese. These forms of protein need to be eaten three times a day within the recommended range of protein intake. That's 3 to 4 ounces three times a day for a woman, and 4 to 5 ounces three times a day for a man.

Unfortunately, it's easy to become overweight eating as a vegetarian. Often a person will eat very small amounts of animal protein or none at all and, in its place, add plenty of starches. In effect, they become more "starcharian" than vegetarian. The net effect is that they keep on gaining weight and losing muscle mass—and end up wondering why such an "inspired" way of eating is making them fat.

Low-glycemic eating is also an inspired way of eating, because it is in alignment with what the body needs to eat for health and proper body-sizing.

Selecting Animal Proteins

As you browse through the meat section of the grocery store, here's what to look for when selecting your protein entrées:

♦ If the seafood is fresh and smells mild, it's a good buy. Avoid fish that's been frozen and thawed, because it has lost flavor and needs to be eaten by the next day.

♦ Stock up on canned or vacuum-packed tuna, sardines, and salmon. These are wild fish, usually processed on ship or right off the ship. Use these for quick meals and snacks.

♦ Shop wisely for price. Buy on sale when the store has a "buy one, get one free" promotion. Meats freeze well.

♦ Keep some frozen hamburger and chicken on hand for the times when you need to whip up a quick meal and you don't want to go to the store.

♦ Purchase lean meats. Trim all visible fat from meats before cooking. This reduces the total amount of saturated fat that you and your family will ultimately eat.

◆ Keep fresh, whole eggs on hand. They'll keep in the refrigerator for several weeks, but most likely, you'll eat them before then. Make boiled eggs so they're handy for snacks or quick meals. They're great to add to tuna-fish salad.

Be sure you have plenty of animal protein in your refrigerator or pantry. That way, you can whip up a quick meal without an extra trip to the store.

The Meat Controversy

Perhaps you've read or heard about the antibiotics and growth hormones added into the feed of livestock. To say the least, it's controversial. No one is sure of the long-term health effects of eating meat raised with these additives.

If you are concerned, purchase "drug-free" meats. They are more expensive, but you may feel that the extra cost is well worth it.

Another controversy about livestock is what it eats. Most livestock are fed grains (mostly corn). But researchers are finding that corn-raised beef is higher in saturated fat and lower in omega-3 essential fatty acids than grass-fed beef. Grass-fed beef is available at natural-food grocery stores and, like the drug-free beef, it costs a little more than grain-fed beef.

Scientists have now discovered that farm-raised salmon contains toxins and contaminants such as polychlorinated biphenyls (PCBs). Additionally, the fish is treated with coloring before being sent to market to make the flesh appear pinkish-red. Farm-raised salmon naturally has a gray color. If you want to avoid eating farm-raised fish, you can purchase wild salmon at stores. Canned salmon and sardines are generally caught in the wild and are either processed on the boat or at the canneries on the coasts.

The Least You Need to Know

◆ Eating moderate amounts of complete protein is essential for your health and for successful glycemic index weight loss.

◆ Only animal protein contains all nine essential amino acids in adequate amounts and is recommended for low-glycemic weight loss.

◆ Eating as a vegan is incompatible with glycemic index weight loss.

◆ Keep your kitchen stocked with a wide variety of animal proteins.

Chapter 12

Dietary Fats

In This Chapter

- ◆ Eating enough fat
- ◆ Avoiding fat-induced insulin resistance
- ◆ Enjoying the benefits of fat for glycemic index weight loss
- ◆ Knowing the importance of essential fatty acids

The word *fat* itself seems fattening. As recently as 10 years ago, some health experts advocated eating only 5 to 10 percent fat in one's daily food intake. Popularly accepted thinking was that eating fat made a person fat, as if it went directly from mouth to thighs and waistline. That thinking is wrong.

Perhaps you followed a low-fat diet for a while and stocked your kitchen with many of the low-fat margarines and salad dressings. If you haven't done so already, you'll be tossing some of these out and visiting the grocery store to purchase some full-fatted products. You'll be shopping for the good fats, such as omega-3s and monounsaturated fats. These types of fats in the right amounts can provide health and weight loss.

Eating the right fats helps you lose weight on a glycemic index weight-loss plan. In this chapter, you learn all about your body's need for fat, which specific types of fat are beneficial for you to eat, and which ones you should avoid.

The Fat-Insulin Resistance Connection

Eating fats is important for losing weight. But eating fat can also be detrimental, depending upon how much and what types of fat you eat. Some types of fats can actually cause insulin resistance. Also, eating 35 percent or more of your calories from fat can cause insulin resistance.

Reducing or eliminating your body's insulin resistance is one of the significant reasons to eat the glycemic index way, so you certainly don't want the types of fat or the amount of fat you eat to lead you back to yet more insulin resistance.

Studies show that two types of fat—saturated fats and trans-fats—cause more insulin resistance compared to other fats.

Saturated Fats

Saturated fats are found in dairy products such as cream, milk, half-and-half, butter, cheese, and ice cream. Saturated fats are also found in meats such as beef, pork, poultry, and lamb.

Glyco Lingo

Saturated fats have a molecular structure that is saturated with hydrogen atoms. Saturated fats are solid at room temperature. Butter and lard are saturated fats.

Thin-spiration

By all means enjoy your steaks and chops, but be smart about it. Remove all visible fat before cooking or grilling. Remove chicken skin before serving. Even small amounts of butter add wonderful flavor to cooked vegetables, so you can still enjoy the taste without slathering your food in it.

Your body can handle some saturated fats just fine. About 10 percent of your food intake can be saturated fat. When you consistently eat more than that amount, insulin resistance can arise. You can also become insulin-resistant if you eat more than 35 percent of your daily calories from fat. A high intake of saturated fats is also linked to heart disease.

Trans-Fatty Acids

Trans-fats are not natural. They were created in the laboratory by modifying other fats. Try to avoid eating trans-fats. They're found in most processed and prepared foods, from cookies and breads to frozen foods and crackers. Margarines, solid vegetable fats, and homogenized peanut butters also contain trans-fats.

One of the problems with regular vegetable oils is that they have a short shelf life. They get rancid rather quickly and don't hold up well to warehousing and shipping. That, plus they're messy. They spill. You can't spread them on bread or crackers. When butter was in short supply during World War II, food manufacturers found that they could take vegetable oils and process them to add more hydrogen molecules. They added some yellow food coloring and—voilà!—they created margarine.

These newly created *trans-fatty acids*, also known as partially hydrogenated vegetable oils or partially hydrogenated oils, were solids at room temperature. They had a long shelf life. They didn't turn rancid easily. Soon manufacturers were selling large tins of white vegetable fat—shortening—that many people preferred over butter for baking. The trans-fats held up well in frying because their flash point was higher than regular vegetable oil. What wasn't to like?

Little did anyone suspect at the time that this hydrogenation process could create so many health problems. Trans-fats have been shown to directly clog arteries and cause heart disease and heart attacks. Today partially hydrogenated vegetable oil is in virtually all the many thousands of processed food items available at the grocery store, at fast-food restaurants, and at fine restaurants. Even French fries are fried in them.

Health experts determined that eating too many trans-fats is bad for the health of your heart. Now we know that eating too many can also bring on insulin resistance. At this time, no reports or studies indicate how much trans-fat is safe to consume, so the National Institutes of Health has essentially recommended that it's best not to eat them at all or in very small quantities.

When you purchase vegetable oils, always purchase *cold-expeller* pressed oils. This guarantees

Glyco Lingo

Trans-fatty acids are fats that have been transformed by adding hydrogen molecules. They are also known as partially hydrogenated oils.

Wrong Weigh

The public health concern over trans-fats is so serious the FDA is requiring that all food manufacturers list the quantity of trans-fatty acids on the nutritional facts label of their products, especially packaged foods, as of January 2006. Many labels already list them. This requirement is prompting food manufacturers to find other safer fats to use.

Glyco Lingo

Cold-expeller pressed oils are extracted from vegetables or nuts without using heat, but only through pressing. When heat is used to extract oils, the heat can damage the oil and trans-fatty acids can be formed.

that they haven't been treated with heat. Oils that are heat-pressed contain small amounts of trans-fats.

Wrong Weigh

Eating a lot of low-fat processed foods can ruin your low-glycemic weight-loss program. How? Because most of these foods, such as spreads, salad dressings, dried mixes, and baked goods, are loaded with high-glycemic carbohydrates, such as sugars, maltodextrins, and modified food starches. By consuming them you may eat less fat, but you're likely to eat a lot more fattening carbs. Instead, eat moderate amounts of real full-fatted foods. When compared to full-fatted dairy, low-fat milk and most low-fat cheeses are not that different in the number of carbohydrate grams, so most are fine to drink and eat.

Good Fats Are Good for You

Eating fat can help you lose weight—that is, when you eat the right amount and types. Your body needs to include monounsaturated fats and polyunsaturated fats. These types of fats contain the highly health-beneficial essential fatty acids.

Glyco Lingo

Monounsaturated fats are dietary fats that are highly beneficial to your health and for losing weight. They are typically liquid at room temperature but solidify when refrigerated.

Monounsaturated Fats

Monounsaturated fats come in totally delicious foods that are good for you. Nutritionists recommend that 10 percent of your daily food intake come from these fats. Health benefits of monounsaturated fats abound and include the following:

Glyco Lingo

LDL is low-density lipoprotein and is considered to be bad cholesterol. Keep your LDL levels below 100 mg/dL. **HDL** is high-density lipoprotein and is considered to be good cholesterol. It's best if your levels of HDL are about 70 to 80 mg/dL and no lower than 35.

- They help reduce insulin resistance.

- They lower blood levels of *LDL*, the so-called "bad cholesterol," without affecting levels of the "good cholesterol," *HDL*.

- They are more chemically stable fats and, as such, may help in protecting against certain cancers, such as breast cancer and colon cancer.

♦ They help support the immune system.

♦ They don't produce inflammatory prostagladins in the body like some fats, so they are protective and help with inflammatory conditions such as rheumatoid arthritis, dementia, diabetes, and heart disease.

♦ In the right amount, they help you lose weight.

Monounsaturated fatty acids, also called omega-9s, are present in larger quantities in the following foods:

♦ Olives

♦ Avocados

♦ Almonds

♦ Hazelnuts

♦ Brazil nuts

♦ Sesame seeds

♦ Cashews

♦ Peanuts

♦ Olive oil

♦ Peanut oil

These food sources either contain no carbohydrates or are extremely low in carbohydrates and are low-glycemic foods. The vegetables and nuts listed above are also high in dietary fiber, except for olives, which contain very little fiber.

Polyunsaturated Fats

The right amount and type of *polyunsaturated fats* are good. And these fats are so important that it's best if you eat 10 percent of your daily food intake from them.

Polyunsaturated fats are divided into two categories: the omega-3 and the omega-6 fatty acids. Omega-3 and omega-6 fats contain the *essential fatty acids*. They are very important for your health and for weight loss.

Essential fatty acids are beneficial for your health and need to be eaten or taken daily for you to realize all their many health benefits.

Glyco Lingo

Polyunsaturated fats are dietary fats with molecules that are not "saturated" with hydrogen atoms due to the presence of two or more double-carbon bonds. Polyunsaturated fats are liquid at room temperature and remain liquid when refrigerated or frozen.

Glyco Lingo

Essential fatty acids (EFAs) are polyunsaturated fats that are essential for your health. They can only be obtained by ingesting them, and hence the government designation "essential." The two main essential fatty acids are alpha-linolenic acid (an omega-3 fatty acid) and linoleic acid (an omega-6 fatty acid).

Ideally, omega-3s and omega-6s should be eaten in the appropriate balance to ensure your good health. In our modern diet, it's easy to eat plenty of omega-6 fats, but not so easy to eat adequate amounts of omega-3 fats. Ideally the balance is one part omega-6s to two parts omega-3s.

Eating Omega-3 Fats

Alpha-linolenic acid (ALA) is metabolized in the body and converted to eicosapentacnoic acid (EPA) and docosahexanenoid acid (DHA). Both of these can be synthesized in the body from alpha-linolenic acid, but they can also be obtained directly from fish and fish oil.

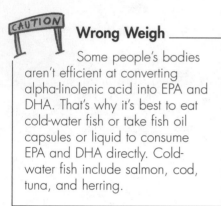

Wrong Weigh

Some people's bodies aren't efficient at converting alpha-linolenic acid into EPA and DHA. That's why it's best to eat cold-water fish or take fish oil capsules or liquid to consume EPA and DHA directly. Cold-water fish include salmon, cod, tuna, and herring.

Here are natural sources of the three types of omega-3 fatty acids:

- Alpha-linolenic acid (ALA). It's found in its highest concentration in fish oils, flaxseeds, and flaxseed oil.

- Eicosapentaenoic acid (EPA). It's best obtained from cold-water fish such as ocean-going salmon, herring, tuna, and cod.

- Docosahexaenoic acid (DHA). It's best obtained from cold-water fish and some algae.

Following are some of the benefits you'll enjoy by eating the omega-3 essential fatty acids:

- They aid the brain neurotransmitters in functioning correctly so that they effectively act as an antidepressant to lift your moods.

- They help support your immune system.

- Of the polyunsaturated fats, the omega-3 fatty acids are especially helpful in reducing inflammation throughout the body, including in joints and skin.

- In some cases, the omega-3 fatty acids can help soothe allergic reactions.

- They assist your body in releasing unneeded stored fat.

- They improve heart health by lowering cholesterol and triglyceride levels.

On your glycemic index weight-loss plan, eat cold-water fish to make sure you receive the full weight-loss and health benefits of these amazing fatty acids. Try to eat three to four servings a week. You can also take fish oil or flaxseed oil supplements. You learn more about supplements in Chapter 16.

Eating Omega-6 Fats

Omega-6s are more common in our modern diet, and you probably already consume adequate amounts. The omega-6s contain the essential fatty acid linoleic acid. Linoleic acid is found in raw seeds and nuts and corn, and sunflower, cottonseed, safflower, and soybean oils.

Gamma-linolenic acid (GLA) is synthesized in your body from the linoleic acid you consume. GLA is considered to be very beneficial, but some parts of the omega-6 fatty acid metabolism produce inflammatory prostaglandins, so, a smaller amount of these fats are recommended. To avoid some of the inflammatory part of the omega-6s, some people prefer to take supplements to be sure they have an adequate amount of the GLA part of the omega-6 fatty acids for cellular metabolism. The GLA part of the omega-6 fatty acid helps with hormone synthesis and more. Some women take supplements of evening primrose oil or borage oil to help reduce menopausal symptoms. Both of these fats contain more GLA than the typical grocery store oils, but the best source of GLA is borage oil, and the second highest source of the GLA is black currant oil.

Omega-6s are widely available in our normal diets; in fact, they may be too widely available. Most people fall short of eating enough omega-3s, which ideally should be eaten in twice the amount as the omega-6s.

Still, the omega-6 fatty acids are valuable, especially the gamma-linolenic acids. It's thought that GLA helps protect against inflammatory conditions such as rheumatoid arthritis, diabetes, and heart disease, to help with nerve transmission, eczema, psoriasis, premenstrual syndrome, and benign breast disease.

Wrong Weigh

Oils such as safflower, soy, corn, cottonseed, and even evening primrose have a lot more of the inflammatory part of the omega-6 fatty acids than borage or black currant oil. Evening primrose oil seems to produce too much inflammation to be used for people with inflammatory conditions, such as rheumatoid arthritis.

Omega-6 foods that are especially high in gamma-linolenic acid include the following:

◆ Borage oil; found in health-food stores.

◆ Black currant oil; found in health-food stores.

Some food sources of omega-6s that have lesser amounts of GLA include the following:

Thin-spiration

For best nutrition, your daily fat intake needs to be about 30 percent of your total food intake divided as follows: one third, or 10 percent each, of monounsaturated fats, polyunsaturated fats, and saturated fats.

◆ Soybean oil

◆ Pumpkin seeds and pumpkin seed oil

◆ Sunflower seeds and sunflower seed oil

◆ Safflower oil

◆ Corn oil

Food sources that are high in saturated fatty acids include butter, palm kernel oil, coconut oil, and red meat. These fats should be eaten in smaller quantities.

The Least You Need to Know

◆ Overeating fat in general, and overeating saturated fats or trans-fats in particular, can increase insulin resistance.

◆ Eat about 30 percent of your food intake as fats—one third each of saturated, monounsaturated, and polyunsaturated fats.

◆ Avoid eating trans-fats, also known as partially hydrogenated vegetable oils.

◆ Eat foods that contain essential fatty acids every day to help you lose weight and to help boost your health.

Dairy

In This Chapter

- ◆ Discovering the uniqueness of dairy products
- ◆ Eating dairy for weight loss
- ◆ Counting dairy carbohydrates
- ◆ Dealing with dairy sensitivity

Some of us just love dairy products. They have been part of our daily diets since childhood, basically from birth! We drank milk as children, we spooned it up with our breakfast cereals, and we all screamed for ice cream. The ice cream man jangled through our childhood neighborhoods on hot summer afternoons and probably still does so.

Dairy products are unique as natural food products. Dairy is the only food that contains significant amounts of these three types of food: animal protein, saturated fats, and carbohydrates. (Hard cheeses, though, contain very few, if any, carbs.)

For someone on a glycemic index weight-loss program, dairy foods can be tricky. Dairy can help with your weight loss, but if you're sensitive to dairy, it can give you some adverse reactions. In this chapter, you learn the complexities of dairy products and how to include dairy in your glycemic index weight-loss program.

The Animal Connection

Dairy stands by itself as a food. It's not easily categorized. Dairy comes from animals and contains substantial healthful protein. In its natural form, it also contains plenty of saturated fat, although you can reduce the fat through low-fat and nonfat versions. Some dairy foods are moderately high in carbs, although some dairy foods have few carbs. When left unsweetened, dairy products are basically low-glycemic foods. Unsweetened dairy products include plain milk, cream, some cheeses, and yogurt.

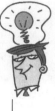

Thin-spiration _____

Most low-fat processed foods have added high-glycemic fillers that can make them off-limits for low-glycemic eaters. But this isn't true for many low-fat dairy products. You can comfortably eat or drink the low-fat varieties of unsweetened dairy products without consuming significantly more carbs than with the full-fat versions. All bets are off on low-fat ice cream, ice milk, and sweetened or artificially sweetened low-fat yogurt, though.

Here's the dairy nutritional scoreboard. Note that the different types of dairy products offer quite different amounts of carbohydrates and saturated fats. All nutrition counts are given in grams.

The dairy nutritional scoreboard includes some surprises. As you can see, one cup of milk contains 12 grams of carbohydrates, almost as many carb grams as a typical slice of bread. Yogurt contains even more carbs, ranging from 12 to 16 grams. The biggest difference is that milk and yogurt are low-glycemic foods with a glycemic load of 3 to 4, whereas white or whole-wheat bread are high-glycemic foods with a glycemic load of 9 to 10.

Dairy Product	Amount	Carbs	GI (Glycemic Index)	GL (Glycemic Load)	Protein	Saturated Fats
Whole milk	1 cup	12	31	4	8	8
2% milk	1 cup	13	32	4	8	5
Skim milk	1 cup	13	32	4	9	0
Cream	2 TB.	1	0	0	0	9
Half-and-half	2 TB.	1	n/a	n/a	1	3
Cottage cheese 4%	1/2 cup	3	n/a	n/a	13	5
Cottage cheese 2%	1/2 cup	4	n/a	n/a	13	3
Cottage cheese (nonfat)	1/2 cup	5	n/a	n/a	13	0
Hard cheese	1 oz.	0	0	0	6	10
Low-fat cheese	1 oz.	1	0	0	8	4.5
Cream cheese	2 TB.	1	0	0	4	20
Cream cheese (light)	2 TB.	2	0	0	3	4.5
Cream cheese (fat-free)	2 TB.	2	0	0	10	0
Whole yogurt (unsweetened)	1 cup	12	36	3	9	10
Yogurt light (unsweetened)	1 cup	16	36	3	10	4
Yogurt (fat-free, unsweetened)	1 cup	16	36	3	10	0
Ice cream (full-fat or premium)	1/2 cup	17	38	5	3	9
Ice cream (light)	1/2 cup	19	50	5	3	4.5
Ice cream (fat-free)	1/2 cup	22	47	5	3	0

Body of Knowledge

Although butter clearly comes from the milk of a cow, it's not considered a dairy product from a nutritional point of view. Instead, butter is categorized as a fat. It contains saturated fat, but no carbohydrates. It's fine to use small amounts of butter, being sure to keep your intake of saturated fat to 10 percent or less of your total fat intake.

High in Saturated Fats

In Chapter 12, you learned that saturated fats need to be eaten in moderation, with preferably only 10 percent of your daily food intake coming from saturated fats. Eating high amounts of saturated fats can increase insulin resistance, the very thing you want your glycemic index weight-loss program to prevent or correct. One way to reduce the amount of saturated fat in dairy is to consume mostly fat-free dairy products or low-fat versions.

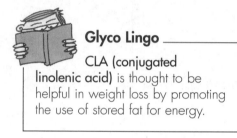

Glyco Lingo

CLA (conjugated linolenic acid) is thought to be helpful in weight loss by promoting the use of stored fat for energy.

Some high-fat dairy products such as butter, cheese, and premium ice cream are good sources of *CLA (conjugated linolenic acid)*. In some studies CLA has been shown to help increase lean muscle mass. Don't overeat high-fat dairy products, but consume them within a balanced diet.

Dairy and Weight Loss

Should you eat dairy products if you're on a glycemic index weight-loss program? Yes, if you tolerate dairy well; no, if you don't.

Some research studies show that consuming dairy products while on a restricted-calorie diet speeds up weight loss and reduces body fat percentage. Some researchers think that the calcium in dairy might be the reason. And, indeed, studies show that the calcium in dairy products seems to promote weight loss.

If you prefer not to eat dairy products or you are allergic to dairy, however, other forms of calcium can help you lose weight. You can get calcium from salmon and sardines, seafood, dark-green leafy vegetables, almonds, asparagus, cabbage, figs, hazelnuts, and calcium supplements.

Calcium is best absorbed in the body when vitamin D, magnesium, vitamin C, vitamin A, some trace minerals, and a sufficient amount of high-quality protein are present. But too much phosphorus, sodium, caffeine, wheat bran, protein, and alcohol can decrease the absorption of calcium.

Calcium absorption is also aided by doing moderate levels of exercise, as you'll be doing on your glycemic index weight-loss program.

Thin-spiration

Some recent nutritional studies suggest that the calcium in dairy products is beneficial for weight loss. But other studies find that calcium from sources other than milk also enhances weight loss. Other sources include salmon or sardines with bones and green leafy vegetables.

Body of Knowledge

Calcium is an important nutrient for more than weight loss. Calcium builds strong bones and teeth and keeps gums healthy. Calcium helps prevent cardiovascular disease by lowering cholesterol levels and blood pressure levels. Calcium aids in brain neurotransmitter regulation and the prevention of muscle cramps. In addition, calcium appears to reduce the risk of colon cancer by binding bile acids and free fatty acids in the colon.

Dairy Sensitivities and Allergies

Dairy is great if you can tolerate it. Perhaps you're one of the many people who don't do well with dairy products. If you experience the following symptoms after eating dairy, then it's best to stop eating dairy products:

- Bloated feeling
- Gas or flatulence
- Phlegm in your throat or head
- Clearing your throat frequently
- Constipation
- Diarrhea

With these kinds of symptoms, you could have a food sensitivity or food allergy to dairy or to the sugar present in milk and yogurt, lactose. Whenever you experience such symptoms, make a record of what foods you ate that may have caused the symptoms. That way, you can pinpoint the offending food.

Wrong Weigh

The most common food allergies are milk, soy, wheat, shellfish, eggs, and peanuts. If you start gaining weight or reach a plateau and you suspect you may have an allergy to one of these foods, stop eating these foods, and you may solve the problem and continue your weight-loss progress. The procedure to more easily detect a food allergy is to stop eating one food at a time, for at least one week. If your symptoms abate, there's a good chance that the food is the cause.

Food allergies can cause mucous buildup throughout the body and within the digestive system. Bloating, gas, and excess phlegm are symptoms of your body's protective reaction to the allergens. Alas, this buildup of mucous also causes weight gain. When you stop eating the offending food, the mucous buildup dissolves and your weight returns to normal.

An allergy to dairy is different from intolerance to dairy products. Most milk intolerances are due to being lactose intolerant. Dairy allergies are associated with reacting to the proteins in the dairy products.

If you have lactose intolerance, you may be able to tolerate dairy by taking a lactase enzyme dietary supplement when eating dairy products. If this works for you, great. If not, don't despair. Many people who can't tolerate high-lactose dairy products such as milk and yogurt can tolerate lower-lactose dairy products such as cottage cheese and hard cheeses. If you can't tolerate dairy, you can still consume calcium in other forms.

Here are other foods that deliver calcium without dairy:

Thin-spiration

To determine whether your calcium supplement breaks down easily for digestion, put the calcium supplement in a glass with 6 ounces of cider vinegar. Stir every 5 minutes. If the tablet or capsule dissolves within 30 minutes, it will dissolve in your stomach.

- Dark-leaf green vegetables, such as kale and spinach.

- Salmon and sardines, with the bones. Canned are great!

- Asparagus, broccoli, cabbage, and other green vegetables.

- Nuts and seeds, such as almonds, filberts, sesame seeds, and flaxseeds.

- Calcium dietary supplements. Take one that breaks down easily and contains magnesium.

The 5 to 10 servings of vegetables and fruits that you're eating daily plus complete protein three times a day provide many of the nutrients that are needed for calcium absorption.

A Healthful Concern

The dairy industry has come under attack in recent years. Nonorganic dairy products are no longer pure, because they contain antibiotics, bovine growth hormone, and other drugs used to enhance milk production. The FDA allows these chemicals to be used in milk production, but questions remain as to their ultimate long-term safety.

If this concerns you, buy organic milk and milk products that are available in health-food stores and in many regular grocery stores.

The Least You Need to Know

- Dairy is the only food group that contains animal protein, saturated fat, and carbohydrates.

- Some dairy products, such as milk, yogurt, and ice cream, can be high in carbs, whereas others, such as hard cheeses, are low carb.

- The calcium in dairy products and other foods helps you lose weight and keep it off.

- If you are sensitive or allergic to dairy, use alternative food sources of calcium plus calcium supplements.

14

Soy

In This Chapter

◆ Getting to know soy

◆ Varying soy varieties

◆ Determining low-glycemic foods with soy

◆ Learning the health concerns of soy

In this chapter, you learn about the different types of soy-based products, how they stack up on the glycemic index, and if they can deliver healthy weight loss. You also learn about what the latest research studies have found about the long-term use of soy-based products.

A Thoroughly Modern Food

Soy products have been touted as an excellent diet food, and many popular diet programs recommend drinking their brand of soy shakes once or twice a day. Most soy shakes are low in fat and have a fair amount of protein, *but* the protein has a low *biological value (BV)*. It sounds as if the soy shakes are great … but. That's a big but.

Although soy was revered as one of the five sacred crops in China over 5,000 years ago, its vast popularity has soared only in the past 30 to 40 years in the

United States. Until recently, people, mostly Asians, ate soy primarily as a green legume, Edamame, or fermented in products such as tofu, natto, tempeh, miso soup, and soy sauce. Soy sauce is a fermented seasoning sauce, or condiment, made from soybeans.

These forms of soy are the most easily digested and assimilated. The fermentation process makes the proteins and other nutrients in soy more bio-available.

One common misconception about soy is that it was a mainstay of the diet for the people of Asia. It wasn't, except perhaps for the poor and underprivileged people or in times of famine. Otherwise, they ate small amounts of soy products, but mostly focused their diets on fish, meat, and vegetables.

> **Glyco Lingo**
>
> **Biological value** or **BV** is a measure of how much nitrogen from the protein is absorbed, retained, and used by the body. This helps determine how much protein the body can actually digest and assimilate from the food. A whole egg is 100, soy is 74.

After World War II, however, the whole nature of soy as a food and agricultural product changed. It became a significant part of agribusiness in the United States. Soy provided an inexpensive source of vegetable protein. It's low in fat and high in some of the amino acids, although not all of them.

Soy contains smaller amounts of two of the nine essential amino acids, *methionine* and *tryptophan*. Soy has a relatively low biological value (BV) of only 74, whereas whey protein has a BV of 104 and a whole egg has a BV of 100. Cow's milk is 91 and beef is 80. Don't plan on using soy-protein products to meet your daily protein needs. They can't.

> **Glyco Lingo**
>
> **Methionine** is one of the nine essential amino acids. It's a powerful antioxidant that neutralizes hydroxyl radicals—one of the most damaging kinds of free radicals. Methionine assists in the breakdown of fats, helps digestion, and plays a role in increasing muscle tone. As you can see, methionine helps you reach some of your weight-loss goals.
>
> **Tryptophan** is a precursor to serotonin in the body. Serotonin is the brain neurotransmitter responsible for feelings of being soothed and uplifted. (Many prescription antidepressants help increase amounts of serotonin in the brain.) Tryptophan plays a role in manufacturing niacin, one of the B vitamins, and it plays a role in the repair of tissues.

In the past 30 years, the number of soy-based products increased dramatically. You can drink soymilk, eat toasted soy nuts, and add soy-protein isolate to your baked goods. Soy shakes are easy to prepare. Just add water to a powdered mix. Soy-based protein bars sit alongside the candy bars at grocery stores and fast-food counters.

Doctors and food manufacturers often recommend soy formulas for infants and soy shakes for oldsters. Vegetarians use soy-based products as a meat substitute. Nutritionists credit the phytoestrogens in soy as being being beneficial for relieving menopausal hot flashes and discomforts.

Glycemic Index of Soy

Soy is classified as a legume—a bean. The basic soybean is low-glycemic, as are most of the foods derived from soy. Following is a sampling of the GI of some low-glycemic, soy-based products:

Low-Glycemic

Toasted soy nuts: 18

Boiled soybeans or Edamame: 18

Soy infant formula: 55

Soymilk: Ranges from 32 to 44

Soy yogurt: 50

Canned soybeans: 14

Tofu hasn't been tested, so for now consider it low-glycemic and in the range of 10 to 20.

Tempeh hasn't been tested, so as for tofu, consider it low-glycemic, at about 10 to 20. *Soy protein isolate* hasn't been tested, but you can estimate it's also in the 10 to 20 range.

Following is a sampling of the GI of a medium-glycemic, soy-based product and a high-glycemic product:

Medium-Glycemic

Soy protein shake mixes that also contain modified food starch, corn syrup solids, sweet whey, maltodextrin, or sugar.

Soymilks with the previously mentioned additives.

Soy protein bars with high-fructose corn syrup, maltodextrin, sugar, or modified food starch.

Power bars: 56

High-Glycemic

Soy protein products that contain food flavor mixes with additives such as those stated previously.

Tofutti frozen dessert: 115

Glyco Lingo

Soy protein isolate is a white powder derived from soybeans through a manufacturing process. This process isolates the protein from other components of the soybean. Soy protein isolate is added to many foods and is a popular ingredient in powdered protein shakes.

If sugar or modified food starch is added to a soy-based product, the glycemic index value rises, as you can tell with the medium-glycemic Power bars and the very high-glycemic Tofutti.

In addition to the additives above, many of these products also contain partially hydrogenated oils (trans-fats), which aren't healthy to eat.

Simply by glancing at this glycemic index information, it seems like soy is great for your weight-loss program. But let's look further at some product characteristics and scientific research.

Limitations

Soy has limitations. And strong critics. Soy products have become controversial as research points to health concerns about eating large quantities of soy-based products. Before you decide how many servings you want to eat per week, you need to learn the concerns about soy and decide for yourself.

◆ Soy has a low biological value, BV, compared to other protein sources, and it doesn't contain all nine essential amino acids in optimal quantities. To obtain a higher-quality protein you need to add animal protein such as meats, eggs, dairy, poultry, whey protein, or fish to your meals.

◆ Most soy products are processed foods, some more than others. Only green soybean Edamame, whole soybeans, and soy sprouts could be considered natural "whole" foods. Soy protein isolate is the most processed. Fermented products such as tempeh, natto, and miso are not as processed and the culturing of these products improves the bioavailability of their nutrients. The isolated protein powders are comparable to other highly processed foods, such as enriched white wheat flour and table sugar. Processed soy-based products contain very little, if any, dietary fiber.

♦ Many people have food sensitivities or allergies to soy. After eating soy, they feel bloated and gassy. These people aren't able to attain adequate digestion and assimilation of this food. If you have this reaction, stop eating soy products.

♦ Soy contains protease inhibitors that make it difficult for your body to break down amino acids. Also, soy contains high levels of phytates and oxalic acid that interfere with the absorption of many nutrients. Protease inhibitors, together with phytates and high levels of oxalic acid, can impair your immune system.

Thin-spiration

Whey protein powder comes from milk and contains all nine essential amino acids in optimal amounts and has a high biological value of 104. You can add whey powder to your soy shakes or you can make shakes with whey powder alone. You'll find whey more beneficial for retaining lean muscle mass than soy protein isolate. Most people find whey easy to digest.

♦ In the concentrated soy-based products, such as tofu, soymilk, and soy protein isolate, the phytoestrogens content is also concentrated. Some menopausal women do experience symptom relief with soy products, but the amount of phytoestrogens consumed may not always be consistent, and because of this, some members of the medical community feel it is not a reliable way to help with hot flashes.

♦ The concentrated protein and isoflavones in soy-based products can adversely affect thyroid functioning, aggravate the thyroid, and may lead to hypothyroidism. This slows metabolism and makes it harder to lose weight.

♦ Long-term studies of people who eat soy-based products frequently show an increased risk of dementia later in life.

♦ Soymilk baby formula may be related to provoking attention deficit disorder, learning disabilities, and behavioral problems in many children.

The final word on the safety of soy hasn't been written. To say the least, however, soy is controversial. If you'd prefer to avoid the controversy altogether, then don't eat or drink soy-based products. If you love soy, then eat it wisely, as described next.

Eating Soy

Any kind of food can be overeaten. Certainly it's easier to overeat treat foods, such as chocolate, donuts, and chips. But there's also another kind of overeating. It comes from thinking that if a little of one food is good for one's health, then more of it is better.

This isn't the case with soy. A little can be good for you. More can possibly be harmful. Our suggestion is, if you are not sensitive to soy, have one serving one to four times a week, and no more. Make soy a small part of your diet and not the main course. If you do choose to eat soy, choose the easier to digest and more nutritious soy products such as Edamame, tempeh, natto, or miso.

From a nutritional point of view, it's best to eat a wide variety of foods and to avoid eating any food repeatedly. Yes, even chocolate.

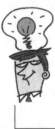

Thin-spiration

A lovely French woman of a certain age who'd been living in the United States for about 20 years commented that a French person wouldn't even consider eating the same food every day or even more than once a week. It astounded her that Americans could eat the same foods, such as burgers and fries, every day. Her common sense approach to nutrition is highly applauded by dietitians.

The Least You Need to Know

- ◆ Soy-based ingredients are present in over two thirds of all manufactured foods.

- ◆ Soy–based products, such as tofu, soymilk, and soy protein isolate, are highly processed forms of soybeans.

- ◆ Soy has a low biological value and contains limited amounts of two essential amino acids, methionine and tryptophan. It doesn't contain the other essential amino acids.

- ◆ Negative health studies on soy make it a controversial food that needs to be eaten infrequently, if at all.

Chapter 15

Sugars and Junk Foods

In This Chapter

- ◆ Identifying junk foods
- ◆ Avoiding sugar and sugar substitutes
- ◆ Reading ingredient lists
- ◆ Shopping for low-glycemic treat foods

Just about everyone loves junk food. This must be true. Otherwise, grocery stores wouldn't devote so much valuable shelf space to fulfilling our country's overwhelming preference for these products.

Look on any high-traffic corner in any city or town in the United States. What do you see? Fast-food establishments that dish up millions of high-glycemic, junk-food meals daily.

We all know these foods are only marginally good for sustaining life and that they offer little, if any, nutritional value or health benefits. Yet junk-food eating goes on and on. Avoiding non-nutritious empty foods can be difficult and exasperating, and it seems that junk food is here to stay. But it doesn't need to stay in your kitchen.

In this chapter, you learn about sugars and the junk ingredients to avoid. As a conscientious consumer of low-glycemic foods, you also need to beware of products that claim to be beneficial to your diet. Many packaged low-carb, low-sugar foods can fool you and aren't the slightest bit good for your weight or your health and aren't necessarily low-glycemic.

The Low-Glycemic Health Concept

Low-glycemic weight-loss programs are specifically designed for you to lose weight. That's their first and primary purpose, and that's why you're reading this book. But the secondary benefit of glycemic index weight-loss is that you can become healthier in general.

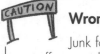

Wrong Weigh

Junk foods and sweeteners offer you almost nothing in terms of nutritional value. They aren't nutrient dense; in fact, they're nutrient devoid.

As you release stored fat, you naturally become healthier as the risk or reality of heart disease, high blood pressure, and diabetes decreases. You're also becoming naturally healthier because you're eating very nutritious foods. As you continue to eat lean meats, good fats, and plenty of vegetables, your body begins to feel great. You have more energy, your skin glows, and overall, eating is simple because you use a clear plan.

The glycemic index weight-loss program highly recommends that you continue eating healthful foods. But plenty of "bad-for-you" foods are often more widely available than the "good-for-you" foods. Here's what you need to know to enjoy the good and avoid the bad. The statements in this list are blanket statements, and you will find exceptions to all of them. But generally speaking, these are what you should avoid:

Glyco Lingo

Mystery ingredients are food package ingredients that you can't pronounce, are ingredients that you can't easily purchase at the grocery store (for example, maltodextrins), or are preservatives and artificial colorings. Avoid purchasing products with more than two or three mystery ingredients, if any.

♦ If the packaging is a fun color and very cute, what's inside is junk food.

♦ If the food has an unnatural color, such as cotton candy, bubble gum, or a blue or chartreuse-colored sports drink, it's junk food.

♦ If the food is in the middle aisles of the grocery store and is at eye level, it's most likely junk food—high in carbs or high in sugar. This isn't always true, so check out the ingredient list.

♦ If the food looks like a candy bar, but claims to be a nutrition bar, approach with caution.

Read the label to be sure it doesn't contain more than two or three *mystery ingredients*. If you want to eat healthy, you should totally avoid eating foods that contain any mystery ingredients.

♦ If your children beg you to buy it for them, most likely it's junk food. We have never yet met a child who begged for string beans.

♦ If it's for sale in a gas station or convenience store, consider it junk food. Only rarely can you find even an apple in a convenience store.

Of course you want to avoid eating junk food; but if you are stranded in the desert or on a mountain top and the only food available is junk food, and you haven't carried any real food with you, and you are about to pass out from hunger, then eat whatever is available—whatever is lowest in sugar and carbs and highest in fiber. Nuts and dried fruit are a good example. Next time, remember to always carry along your own treats and snacks.

> **CAUTION**
>
> **Wrong Weigh**
>
> Steer clear of most packaged foods labeled low fat. Usually they're high in carbohydrates. Instead, choose the full-fat versions of salad dressings, mayonnaise, and spreads. To avoid consuming too many calories from these higher fat products, eat small portions.

Sugar, Plus Variations

To tell the honest truth without any bias toward what's healthful, sugar simply tastes wonderful. In a sense, it doesn't actually taste like anything other than utter sweetness. Sugar has a mystery all its own. Part of the mystery is its overwhelming allure; part is how something that tastes so divine can be so bad for us. It doesn't seem fair.

Now that nutritionists and health-food gurus know the downside of sugar, many millions of research dollars have been poured into finding a sweet-tasting substitute. Ideally, the substitute would be better than neutral for your health—it would actually be good for you. So far, those millions haven't found the sweet fountain of great taste and great health. The search continues.

Any sweetener, whether natural or artificial, is thought to cause a beta-endorphin increase in your body that stimulates sugar cravings, so it's best to use all sweeteners sparingly. But until the time when a really great substitute is created or discovered, here's the lowdown on available sweeteners:

◆ **Table sugar, or sucrose.** Many people are sensitive to sugar. Just 1 teaspoon contains 4 grams of carbohydrates, 15 calories, a glycemic index of 61, and a glycemic load of 2.5. Sugar can be acceptable in small amounts if eaten infrequently and with other foods to keep the glycemic load low.

◆ **Natural cane sugar.** This is sucrose sprayed with brown coloring. It has the same stats as table sugar.

◆ **Brown sugar.** This is also sucrose sprayed with brown coloring. It has the same stats as table sugar. Usually brown sugar is a darker brown color than natural cane sugar.

◆ **Evaporated cane syrup.** This ingredient appears on labels for foods that are sold at health-food stores. Beware. This is simply a fancy and healthy-sounding name for table sugar, also known as sucrose.

◆ **Fructose.** The sugar found in fruits. Good for you when eaten in fruits. Not so good when overeaten. This could mean eating too much fruit at one time, drinking a large glass of fruit juice, drinking or eating foods sweetened with high-fructose corn syrup, or using too much packaged fructose crystals as a sweetener in foods. Has been shown to raise triglyceride levels. Just 1 teaspoon has 4 grams of carbohydrates, 15 calories, a glycemic index of 19, and a glycemic load of 1.

◆ **High-fructose corn syrup.** Used in many processed foods, including sodas. This is a highly controversial product. It is made from genetically modified corn. A teaspoon contains 5 grams of carbohydrates and 20 calories; the glycemic index and glycemic load are unavailable. Avoid this product.

◆ **Agave nectar.** Made from agave cactus. Available at health-food stores. A teaspoon contains 5 grams carbs, 16 calories, a glycemic index of 10, and a glycemic load of 1. This has more nutrients than table sugar, but is still high in carbs.

◆ **Honey.** Naturally occurring—even the caveman and cavewoman ate honey. It's the only paleo food that contains a very dense form of carbohydrates. A teaspoon contains 6 grams of carbs, 20 calories, a glycemic index of 55, and a glycemic load of 3. Honey gives you some unique nutritional benefits. It can be helpful for people who suffer from seasonal allergies, and it contains small amounts of minerals and B vitamins. It is not advised for people who want to keep insulin levels low.

♦ **Other syrups, such as rice syrup and barley syrup.** Contain carbohydrates and calories similar to corn syrup. This is not recommended.

♦ **Sugar alcohols.** Also called polyols. Some, such as mannitol, are used in making sugarless candies. Don't be fooled. Sugar alcohols still have calories. They don't lift blood sugar levels, but instead are incompletely absorbed into the bloodstream. Chemically, sugar alcohols aren't sugar, so food manufacturers can claim their products are sugar-free. One big drawback is that eating them can cause flatulence and diarrhea. Common sugar alcohols include mannitol, sorbitol, xylitol, lactitol, isomalt, maltitol, and hydrogenated starch hydrolysates. Manitol, sorbitol, and xylitol occur naturally in fruits and vegetables.

♦ **Aspartame, also known as Equal, is an artificial sweetener.** Aspartame is non-nutritive and is approved as safe by the FDA. It is used widely as an ingredient in diet sodas and thousands of other processed foods, such as sugarless yogurt, popsicles, and lemonade. Some research studies conducted since FDA approval indicate that aspartame may not be safe. Because its safety is in question and a vigorous controversy continues, we can't recommend aspartame. Eating aspartame could stall any weight-loss program and is thought to increase beta-endorphin production, which triggers sweet cravings.

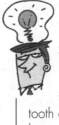

Thin-spiration

If you have seasonal airborne allergies and would like to use bee products for nutritional support, use bee pollen rather than honey. Bee pollen has virtually no carbohydrates but plenty of B vitamins. Take a very small amount at first, as it can cause an allergic reaction. If bee pollen suits you, you can take up to one teaspoon a day.

Thin-spiration

Unlike other sugar alcohols, xylitol can offer some health benefits because it isn't fermented by oral bacteria, so it doesn't cause tooth decay, and xylitol inhibits bacterial growth.

♦ **Sucralose, also known as Splenda, is an artificial sweetener.** It's derived through chemically altering table sugar by adding chlorine molecules. Sucralose is 600 times sweeter than table sugar and doesn't raise blood sugar and insulin levels. The FDA has approved it as a sugar substitute, but, as in the case of aspartame, new research indicates that long-term use could present health problems. Many people like sucralose, but we can't wholeheartedly recommend it.

Glyco Lingo

Fruit ogliosaccharides are a probiotic nutritional supplement that selectively nourishes the friendly bacteria in the intestines. This increases the number of good bacteria in your gut. Not only is stevia safe, FOSes are definitely good for you.

◆ **Stevia with FOS is not an artificial sweetener, but rather a totally natural product.** Stevia is an herb from South America that is considered safe and without side effects. It's 300 times sweeter than sugar. When combined with FOS—*fruit ogliosaccharides*—it has a smoother taste and is 10 times sweeter than sugar. The FDA hasn't approved stevia for use as a sweetener, but it's widely available at grocery stores and health-food stores. We highly recommend stevia with FOS as a sweetener. Its glycemic index is 0. Just ¼ teaspoon, which is very sweet, has less than 1 gram of carbohydrates. You can also use plain stevia as a sweetener, if you like.

Junk-Food Ingredients

We doubt that food manufacturers set out to purposely invent the next junk food. Instead, they attempt to create foods that people will want to eat. These are foods that taste so good that people are compelled to purchase them over and over again. In essence, they're selling calories, and the population as a whole loves high-carbohydrate calories wrapped in exciting packaging with fun colors and containing virtually no nutritional value.

But what's in the package or what's not in the package makes the most difference to you and your weight-loss success. Some foods are high in carbs, whereas others can undermine your glycemic index weight-loss efforts. So here's a list of ingredients you want to avoid.

◆ **White flour.** Also known as enriched, made from whole grains, fortified, and sometimes labeled natural. Instead, choose products that list whole-grain ingredients.

◆ **Fruit drinks.** Usually sweetened with high-fructose corn syrup or other sugars, such as evaporated cane sugar. These are filled with sugar and offer very little real fruit.

◆ **Fruit juice.** A highly concentrated form of fruit without any of the beneficial dietary fiber. You're better off eating real fruit.

- ◆ **Food starch.** Fillers such as maltodextrins and modified food starches are high-glycemic and high in calories.

- ◆ **Partially hydrogenated vegetable oil or partially hydrogenated oils.** These are trans-fats, which should always be avoided.

- ◆ **Artificial coloring.** A non-nutritive chemical that only adds color, and could cause a reaction in some sensitive individuals.

- ◆ **Preservatives.** Used to extend product shelf life, and not usually considered beneficial.

- ◆ **Monosodium glutamate, or MSG.** Used as a flavor enhancer, it actually mimics the taste of proteins, which is why it's often added to foods such as soups, bouillon, and packaged meat products. MSG is known to cause headaches and discomfort in some people.

- ◆ **Olestra.** Used to substitute for fat and can cause upset stomach. Many food manufacturers are no longer using this product because of undesirable side effects.

- ◆ **Fried foods.** At this writing, fried foods are always fried in partially hydrogenated vegetable oils. This includes French fries and onion rings, as well as fried chicken and fish fillets. Additionally, the coating on the chicken and fish is usually made from white flour.

- ◆ **Dough tenderizers and other odd ingredients.** If it simply doesn't make sense to you, pass on it.

You can usually find some high-quality packaged food items at health-food stores and in some grocery stores in the health-food section. However, continue to read labels, because even totally organic foods can be junk foods. Organic lemonade sweetened with organic evaporated cane syrup is junk food. Organic evaporated cane syrup is another way of saying table sugar.

The Low-Carb Shelf

Grocery stores are stocking more and more low-carb processed foods as consumers continue to realize the benefits of eating the low-carb way. But beware! Low-carb doesn't necessarily mean low-glycemic, or that you're eating a healthy food.

You need to read the ingredients. Look for foods that contain few preservatives and no high-glycemic ingredients, such as enriched wheat and high-fructose corn syrup or other sweeteners. Also, make sure the ingredients are everyday foods, and not such things as modified food starches and partially hydrogenated vegetable oils. The best place to find high-quality and highly nutritive low-glycemic foods is on the outside perimeter of the grocery store. There you'll find vegetables, fruit, meats, and fish. You absolutely can't go wrong eating the basic foods of glycemic index weight loss.

The Least You Need to Know

- ◆ Eating junk foods is incompatible with eating for glycemic index weight loss.

- ◆ Eating healthful, nutrient-dense foods ensures your weight-loss success and boosts your health.

- ◆ Use sugars and sweeteners sparingly to prevent cravings and avoid nutritionally devoid carbohydrates.

- ◆ Carefully read low-carb packaged food labels; not all of them are healthful.

Chapter 16

Nutritional Supplementation

In This Chapter

- ◆ Improving your digestion and assimilation
- ◆ Unwinding stress with B vitamins
- ◆ Using minerals to manage insulin resistance
- ◆ Keeping your electrolytes balanced

Taking one-a-day or two-a-day or maybe even more-a-day vitamins and supplements can make glycemic index weight loss happen faster. When your body is missing or is low on some important nutrients, your weight-loss efforts can stall.

That's not to say that simply by taking the right mix of nutritional supplements you can lose all the weight without reducing your food intake. That won't happen. But combining the two may prove a great solution. Eating the glycemic way and using nutritional supplements that support your body together will help you release stored fat. In fact, you can make up for lost or missing nutrients from when you were eating fewer healthful foods.

The Need for Supplements

Controversies about nutritional supplementation have raged for years. One side asserts that all the vitamins and minerals that people need can be assimilated from the food they eat. The other side strongly suggests that, although that was once true in the good old days, it's no longer true today.

You know which side is winning. Just look up the number of health-food stores in your phone book, or visit the nutritional-supplement section of any grocery store, drugstore, or discount chain. People buy supplements and plenty of them.

In the good old days, fruits and vegetables were picked ripe and eaten within hours. Food animals grazed freely on grassy plains. Fish were caught fresh from streams, lakes, and oceans and eaten soon afterward. "Junk" was something people threw away, not something they ate joyously and eagerly. In short, during those good old days, food contained more nutritional value than it does today.

Obviously you can live without taking nutritional supplements. But we don't know why you would want to. All evidence points to people living better and healthier lives with a little help from health-food stores. Health practitioners and doctors are now widely recommending that their patients take nutritional supplements.

Losing weight is challenging. And a little or even a lot of help along the way is available to you in health-food stores, drugstores, or discount chain stores.

In the United States, the FDA does not consistently enforce quality standards for dietary supplements. Supplement manufacturers aren't required to test their products to verify that they contain standard and consistent amounts of natural herbs, minerals, and vitamins. As a result, consumers may consume varying amounts of an herb or vitamin with each bottle they purchase. The products can also contain filler ingredients, which could cause allergic reactions in some people. Here are some guidelines to help you purchase safe and effective products:

◆ Buy only commercially sold products from reliable sources. The label should include a list of the ingredients in detail. Look for the GMP (Good Manufacturing Processes) stamp of approval. To have this stamp is optional, but it does mean that the company is inspected and goes through safe and reliable manufacturing methods and that they list all ingredients on the label as well as the specific amounts of these ingredients.

◆ Buy standardized extracts whenever possible. This provides you with some assurance that the active ingredient is present in the amounts you want and expect.

- Purchase supplements and use them before the expiration date. Store all supplements in a cool, dry place. If the supplement requires refrigeration, be sure to refrigerate.

- Don't buy supplements that contain excessive doses of trace minerals. High doses of one mineral can offset the benefits of another. For example, too much zinc can interfere with the absorption of copper.

Following are some guidelines for optimizing the use of supplements:

- Take most supplements with or immediately after a meal. The digestive enzymes and hydrochloric acid excreted when you eat help break down not only the nutrients in the food, but also those in the supplements.

- Some supplements, such as some of the amino acids taken for a specific purpose, need to be taken on an empty stomach. If the label doesn't provide this information, ask your dietitian, nutritionist, or physician.

- Take one new product at a time. If the product is causing adverse reactions, it can be easier to detect and pinpoint this way.

- Some natural remedies contain potent chemicals that can interfere with absorption or other medicines you might be taking. Talk to your pharmacist or doctor to check on drug-supplement interactions. You can often find this information online as well. Your need for specific supplements can change from time to time, so once or twice a year evaluate which supplements you're taking. Make changes if it seems necessary. If you take a lot of tablets or capsules, you may be able to consolidate some or possibly eliminate them from your daily regimen.

Your Digestion and Assimilation

The first place to start when you consider nutritional supplementation isn't with a vitamin pill. Instead, the place to start is with your body's digestion and assimilation mechanisms. You can be taking the most expensive and powerful vitamin and mineral supplement in the world, but if your digestion and assimilation processes aren't working well, your body isn't going to realize the benefits.

Digestion is a very complicated process. To digest your food well, you need to have your digestive enzymes functioning well, and you need an adequate amount of hydrochloric acid to be present in your stomach. Very frequently, by the time a person reaches 35 years old, digestion becomes less efficient. The person isn't receiving the full nutritional value of the foods he or she eats. Given that many foods people eat are already low in nutrients, such as junk foods, the body isn't receiving enough value from the foods eaten.

Digestive Enzymes

Stress can cause havoc with digestion. Many of us react to stress by not adequately producing digestive enzymes. In addition, age also can decrease our ability to produce hydrochloric acid and digestive enzymes. Taking digestive enzyme supplements is a boon to virtually everyone over the age of 40, and maybe even for some younger people. They can help your body receive nutritional value from the foods you do eat, and they can help your body digest the nutritional supplements you're going to take.

Body of Knowledge

People with cystic fibrosis, celiac disease, and Crohn's disease have an important need for pancreatic enzymes that the body does not make on its own. The rest of us can use digestive enzymes to aid with our digestion. Symptoms of indigestion include bloating, belching, abdominal pain, and excess gas.

Wrong Weigh

You've seen or read many ads and commercials for products to remedy indigestion, constipation, or diarrhea. Most likely, you've used them just as millions of other people have. You may not have realized it then, but your digestion and assimilation wasn't working well when you took them.

Most individuals with indigestion of any degree can benefit from digestive enzyme supplements with hydrochloric acid. Look for the following components:

- Hydrochloric acid (HCl), often formulated as betaine hydrochloride, or HCl betaine is advised. Hydrochloric acid helps stimulate the pancreas to create enzymes that digest proteins. Some people may not secrete adequate amounts of hydrochloric acid to digest protein well. You only need HCl with meals that contain protein. But as you eat a lower glycemic diet, your meals will contain protein for each meal, and it may benefit you to take it at all meals.

- Enzymes that digest protein include bromelain, pepsin, papain, or protease. These work hand in hand with the hydrochloric betaine above.

- Lipase is an enzyme that digests fat.

- An enzyme that digests carbohydrates will be useful now that you're eating complex carbs such as vegetables and whole grains. The enzymes that digest carbs are amylase or invertase.

Many digestive enzyme products available at the store assist with digesting proteins, fats, and carbohydrates. However, be aware that a number of studies have shown that gastric acid may inactivate most, if not all, the pancreatic enzyme preparations. If you choose to use digestive enzymes, using them after eating may be more beneficial. In people who have gastric hyposecretion of HCL, enzyme substitution can be administered as granules to enable mixing and simultaneous transport of enzymes with the food already eaten. If you have gastric hyposecretion of HCL and choose to only take HCL, and not digestive enzymes, the HCL should be taken with or immediately before eating foods with protein.

> **Thin-spiration**
>
> If you have weak or splitting fingernails, you may find that they become stronger within a month of taking hydrochloric betaine with meals. Your nails are made of protein, and now your body will be better able to assimilate the protein you eat.

Try one. Then, if for any reason you don't like the results, select a different brand or formulation until you find the one that works best with your body. Most products on the market are not that potent and will not cause a lot of problems if you don't need them; however, if you take excessive doses of pancreatic enzymes, it may result in gastrointestinal adverse effects, such as nausea, vomiting, diarrhea, and abdominal cramps.

If you have difficulty with digestion, keep trying. There's a digestive aide that can work well for you, and there are other ways described next that can help.

Herbs

Herbs that may help stimulate the body's ability to better secrete digestive enzymes include gentian, bitter melon, dandelion, horehound, prickly ash, and artichoke.

Herbs that may help relieve symptoms of indigestion, especially when there is excessive gas, include anise, basil, caraway, cinnamon, cloves, fennel, dill, sage, thyme, turmeric, and lemon balm.

Herbs that help treat indigestion and heartburn include ginger, licorice, and slippery elm.

Fiber

By eating a low-glycemic diet, you will automatically be getting a good amount of fiber; however, a fiber supplement might still be needed in some cases.

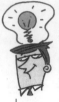

Thin-spiration _____

Here are some other ways you can enhance the digestion and absorption of the nutrients in foods and in supplements: Eat smaller portions at each meal. (For instance, a smaller portion of protein will be easier to digest.) Eat in a relaxed atmosphere. Stress and eating on the run can cause a decrease in the body's ability to secrete HCL and digestive enzymes. You can also eat a bitter or sour type of food or seasoning at the beginning of a meal. Examples of this include bitters, endive, lemon, limes, and vinegar. When you chew your food thoroughly and eat slowly, you also improve digestion and assimilation.

Fiber supports your entire digestive and assimilation function. Most people eat fewer than 15 grams of fiber a day. But a person needs 25 to 50 grams of dietary fiber every day to have regular elimination and increase food transit time through the body. You can't expect to lose weight if you aren't having at least daily bowel movements.

Fiber has other benefits:

♦ Fiber absorbs toxins and allergens from food and transports them quickly through the body.

♦ Fiber gives you a feeling of satiation when eating. Basically, fiber fills you up and the full feeling reduces your desire to overeat.

♦ Fiber slows the absorption of sugars and starches in the stomach, thus helping you avoid hyperinsulinism.

♦ Fiber helps reduce or eliminate both diarrhea and constipation.

♦ A high-fiber diet can help prevent colon cancer and other colon and digestive disorders.

♦ Fiber helps lower blood cholesterol and triglyceride levels, and may also reduce the risk of developing gallstones.

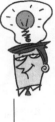

Thin-spiration _____

Robin was 70 pounds overweight. She was only having one bowel movement every two to three weeks. No wonder she couldn't lose weight. Her body was holding on to everything she ate. Robin experienced painful backaches due to the backup of waste products in her bowels. Fortunately, fiber supplements worked for her, and her glycemic index weight-loss program began to work. She finally lost weight.

The easiest, healthiest, and least-expensive way to take fiber is to consume psyllium. You can purchase psyllium in large bulk bags at health-food stores. It's unsweetened and unflavored, so it has no taste. Mix a heaping tablespoon of psyllium in a glass of water and drink quickly, before it starts to gel. Follow with another glass of water. Each heaping tablespoon contains about 7 grams of fiber and no carbohydrates or calories.

Good times to take psyllium are when you awaken before breakfast or just before bed. You can also take psyllium before or after a meal. Don't take fiber supplements at the same time you take medications or other nutritional supplements. The fiber could absorb them and diminish their effectiveness.

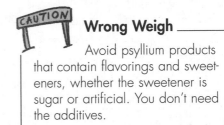

Wrong Weigh

Avoid psyllium products that contain flavorings and sweeteners, whether the sweetener is sugar or artificial. You don't need the additives.

The Good Bacteria

Your digestive supplementation should also include intestinal support so that your body can efficiently assimilate the nutrients from your food. To do that, you need good bacteria in your intestines. This is especially important after taking an antibiotic medication. Here's what the good bacteria does:

♦ Produces some B vitamins. B vitamins are important for all bodily metabolic processes, and they also help reduce stress. As you know, plenty of overeating is prompted by stress.

♦ Competes in the gastrointestinal tract with the pathogenic organisms, thus protecting us from harmful pathogenic by-products.

♦ Functions as an antifungal. It helps reduce yeast infections as well as other fungal infections.

♦ Enhances the absorption of nutrients.

If you don't have enough good bacteria in your intestines, you may experience gas, bloating, constipation, malabsorption of nutrients, and perhaps candida overgrowth (also known as a yeast infection).

Thin-spiration

Good bacteria thrive on fruit ogliosaccharides (FOS), which are present in vegetables and fruits, as well as in the natural sweetener, stevia with FOS. What a great reason to eat your veggies and enjoy the sweet taste of stevia with FOS.

Good bacteria are lactobacillus and bifidobacterium bacteria. You can purchase both in pill, capsule, or powder form. Most brands need to be kept refrigerated. If you travel frequently or find it inconvenient to keep the supplements refrigerated, you can find a version that doesn't require refrigeration.

You can take the good bacteria supplements up to three times a day, preferably at times away from meals, and definitely away from when you take fiber supplements. Take one to two capsules or tablets one to three times a day.

Now that your digestion and assimilation are in good working order, it's time to start taking additional supplements for nutritional support.

Vitamins and Minerals

You need a powerful vitamin and mineral supplement that contains all the basics including the following:

Thin-spiration

You can take B vitamins sublingually, meaning under your tongue, by taking a liquid version. This delivery method bypasses your stomach and digestive system entirely. Instead, the B vitamins are absorbed through the mucous membranes of your mouth. You can find liquid B vitamins at the health-food store. You can also use them when you feel highly stressed or need quick energy.

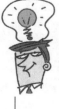

Thin-spiration

In a study done by the University of Pretoria in South Africa, vitamin C helped combat stress by lowering cortisol levels by up to 30 percent.

- The B vitamins. Some of these are the hardest to digest and assimilate, but now that your digestion is in tip-top shape, your body can benefit from taking B vitamins as a nutritional supplement. Because B vitamins are water soluble, unused portions are flushed from the body daily—so you need to replenish them daily.

  B vitamins are used up quickly when you're stressed, and the mere fact of being on a weight-loss plan is stressful. And that's not counting what else is going on in your life. Take a B-vitamin formulation made specifically for high stress. Take one per day or follow the label guidelines, if different.

- Vitamin C is important as an antioxidant, and it's required for at least 300 metabolic functions in the body. Take up to 1000 mg a day.

- Vitamin E in its natural form helps balance hormones and helps prevent free radical damage due to excess oxidation that can occur with both excess weight and during weight loss. Also, vitamin E helps prevent the oxidation of the unsaturated fats that contain the essential fatty acids. Take 200 to 800 IUs a day.

♦ Calcium. Low calcium levels can increase the stress hormone cortisol's ability to generate stress-related fat. Calcium can help burn fat by decreasing levels of lipoprotein lipase, a fat-storing enzyme. Several studies show that inadequate calcium in the diet is related to weight gain. The RDA (Recommended Daily Amount) for calcium is 800 mg, but if you're a woman over age 35, recommended levels go up to as high as 1500 mg per day.

♦ Magnesium is depleted when a person is insulin-resistant or has hyperinsulinism. But magnesium also helps the body use insulin effectively and safely. You also need magnesium to avoid muscle cramps and to soothe nerves. Take a magnesium supplement starting with 250 mg a day on up to 750 mg a day. Take magnesium to improve bowel tolerance. If you develop diarrhea, cut back the amount of magnesium until your stools are normal. In general, the amount of magnesium you take should equal one half the amount of calcium you consume.

♦ Chromium assists the cells in uptaking insulin, so it aids you with eating the low-glycemic way and keeping your insulin levels low. Chromium helps build muscle, decrease body fat, and lower cholesterol levels. Take between 300 to 800 mcg per day. Start with a smaller dosage and increase it if you need more.

♦ Vanadium helps body cells absorb blood sugar more effectively, thus reducing insulin resistance. There is no RDA for vanadium, but nutritionists recommend you take between 40 to 100 mcg a day. Most people only require 40 mcg, but if you already have diabetes, you could benefit from taking more. If you prefer not to take a supplement, foods that are high in vanadium include black pepper, shellfish, parsley, and mushrooms.

♦ Selenium helps enhance the action of vitamin E as an antioxidant and is thought to help in the prevention of diabetes. Take 30 mcg a day.

Some vitamin/mineral products are formulated specifically for persons who are diabetic, who have insulin resistance, or who are eating the low-glycemic way. Check out those first before you purchase several bottles of supplements. It's obviously easier to take 1 or 2 capsules or tablets a day as opposed to 10 or 20. But overall, it's quite important to take the supplements you need for health and weight loss. If you're going to commit your energy to eating a low-glycemic diet, you want to give yourself every opportunity to succeed. The right supplements make it easier.

The Good Fats

Your body needs essential fatty acids (EFAs) every day, not just to facilitate weight loss but to also enable you to feel your best. These important fats actually let you release stored fat. But they do far more than that. EFAs keep your moods elevated and keep your joints and muscles in good working order.

Thin-spiration

The more you eat junk foods and highly processed foods that contain omega-6 polyunsaturated fats and partially hydrogenated vegetable oils (trans-fatty acids), the more good fats you need to consume to keep your body healthy and in balance.

Take from 1 teaspoon to 1–2 tablespoons of an essential fatty acid liquid once a day. This can be flaxseed oil or a combination of plant and animal oils. Or take 4 to 12 capsules of fish oil a day.

You can also eat cold-water fish, such as salmon, cod, herring, and sardines three or more times a week in place of taking supplements. Or take the supplements *and* eat the cold-water fish. Just make sure you eat plenty of essential fatty acids.

Helpful Supplements

In special circumstances, the following supplements are highly beneficial for weight loss. Whether you will need them depends on the state of your body and your health:

◆ Electrolytes are great for cellular replenishment after exercise, sweating, or stress. They keep your body hydrated. Electrolytes are mineral complexes of potassium, magnesium, sodium, and calcium. Electrolytes can also give you a quick energy boost after a long day spent driving or sitting in meetings. Avoid using electrolyte beverages that contain sugars, high-fructose corn syrup, or artificial sweeteners. Instead, use electrolyte powders you mix with water. Our favorite brand is Emergen-C. You can find boxes of Emergen-C at health-food stores and grocery stores. It's great-tasting, too.

Wrong Weigh

If you have repeated or continual yeast infections, chances are good you find it impossible to lose weight. Most yeast infection remedies and diets aren't very effective. A yeast-free diet is grueling and not effective if your body stays acidic. Try a greens drink. You'll likely love the results.

◆ "Greens" drinks are wonderful at killing off candida and yeast overgrowth conditions. Yeast can't live in an alkaline environment. They need your body to be acidic. Greens drinks are actually powders made from all sorts of vegetables. You mix a tablespoon in a glass of water and drink it down. Usually 1 or 2 tablespoons a day are plenty to rid your body of a yeast overgrowth condition. Then simply drink a glass of greens several times during the week to keep your body in a slightly alkaline state, which will keep those yucky yeasties at bay. Overall, greens drinks are very healthy for you and provide you with many phytonutrients, antioxidants, vitamins, and minerals.

Thin-spiration

When you feel your body needs a restorative tonic after several days or longer of travel, vacation, business meetings, or illness, try taking a greens drink for a couple days. Chances are good the tonic will refresh your body and rebalance your energy.

Supplements to Avoid

Beware of quirky supplements that promise you a simple, easy way to enjoy weight loss. Simple weight loss simply doesn't exist. Here's a list of some questionable products or ingredients that are currently highly promoted.

♦ **Bitter orange.** Bitter orange sounds safe enough. It's extracted from Seville oranges, the ones from which orange marmalade is made. It sounds safe enough, and it is in very small, naturally occurring quantities. But the extract is full of amphetamine-type stimulants that artificially boost your metabolism. You could lose weight and stored fat quickly. Then you'll experience the rebound effect and gain the weight all over again.

You probably remember bitter orange's cousin, ephedra, that's now banned in the United States by the FDA. Bitter orange, also known as citrus aurantium, is on the watch list of the FDA. They've had plenty of reports that it's not safe.

Most commercially advertised weight-loss pills contain bitter orange. Pass on it.

♦ **Carb blockers.** These sound as if they would be wonderful. A person could eat a dozen donuts and not digest the carbs. This reasoning is flawed. Carb blockers are basically a form of dietary fiber that absorbs some of the sugar and starch from foods you eat and prevents them from being absorbed.

You could take carb blockers, but you can do just as well by eating foods high in fiber and using a fiber supplement such as psyllium. On a glycemic index

Wrong Weigh

Fat blockers can't distinguish between fat from French fries and the good fats that are essential for your health. In addition, fat blockers decrease the absorption of fat-soluble vitamins such as vitamin E. You don't need to spend money on fat blockers. Instead, use the money to purchase good fats supplements and fresh vegetables.

weight-loss program, you are eating nutritionally important and healthy carbohydrates, so you don't need to block their absorption.

- **Fat blockers.** Fat blockers are actually prescription medications that block fat absorption. They haven't been proven effective for long-term weight loss. The side effects, such as bowel leakage, are pretty disgusting. Pass on anything that could be embarrassing.

If any other "miracle" weight-loss supplements come your way, check out the fine print.

The Least You Need to Know

- Put your digestion and assimilation in tip-top working order to receive the utmost benefit from foods and supplements.

- Vitamins and minerals give your body support for blood sugar and insulin regulation as well as for weight loss.

- Use greens drinks to kill off yeast infections that otherwise can prevent weight loss.

- Avoid supplements that promise you'll lose weight.

Part 4

Eating for All Occasions

Eating under any circumstances can be just as much fun and just as delicious when you eat based on the glycemic index. Don't be afraid of parties, family get-togethers, and potlucks after you learn how to navigate the buffet table. You can always contribute a dish of delicious low-glycemic food to the gathering. Grocery shopping requires that you learn new patterns and skills. Learn what aisles and sections to frequent and which ones to avoid. Cooking meals based on the glycemic index for yourself and the entire family can be easy when you remember to focus on "meats and vegetables" with flourishes and variety.

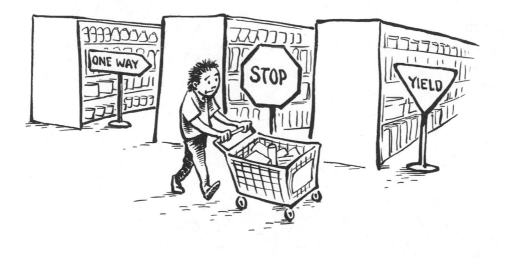

Chapter 17

Eating a Meal or a Snack

In This Chapter

◆ Savoring low-glycemic foods

◆ Eating without stress

◆ Creating a soothing eating environment

◆ Appreciating snacks

Eating is a requirement of life. You need to eat. As you've figured out by now, there's no way you can avoid eating. You need to eat to survive, and if you're like most people, you need to eat at least three times a day and perhaps more, especially if you like to snack.

Fortunately for us, in addition to being a requirement, eating is highly pleasurable. We like to eat. Food tastes good and food appeals to our senses of sight, smell, and taste. We even stimulate our sense of touch when we eat with our fingers, handle food in the kitchen, and chew and swallow.

You already know how to eat, but do you know how to get the utmost pleasure from your food and the process of eating? You might find that as you derive more pleasure from eating, you are satisfied with less food. In this chapter, you learn the sensuous way to eat a meal or a snack so that all your senses feel satisfied.

Love the Food You're With

To use a line (modified for our purposes) from an old song, "If you can't be with the food you love, then love the food you're with." Adopting that attitude as you eat the low-glycemic way can make your meals a lot more fun.

In the past, dieting and food restriction may have meant boring and unpleasant meal-times. You may have found your food choices limited and unpalatable, or you may have watched the rest of your family members wolfing down the foods you craved while you were left sitting with Melba toast and a thin slice of cheese.

To succeed in eating based on the glycemic index, mealtimes need to change for the better. So start telling yourself that you love vegetables and salads. Lean meats make your mouth water. Essential fatty acids are yummy. (Okay, that may be going a bit too far.)

After all, what are your choices?

- To feel deprived, fat, and angry
- To apologize to everyone you dine with because you need to eat differently than everyone else
- To explain in intimate detail all about your new glycemic index weight-loss plan
- To grunt like a caveman or cavewoman and eagerly eye your meat and vegetables
- To eat with joy and gratitude that glycemic index weight loss is working for you

The best choices are obvious, but perhaps not the easiest (although grunting as a paleo person can be fun in the appropriate setting).

Setting the Mood

Realistically, you're a busy person. Your time matters to you. You eat lunch in between answering the phone and managing your e-mail or in between meetings, carpools, and running errands. Your life is busy, and your meals are mostly rushed. It's easy just to grab something convenient and quick to eat, which could be part of the reason you're on a program to lose weight. This method of eating isn't working and it is definitely fattening.

Being busy when you are eating is certainly not sensuous and pleasurable. It increases anxiety and worsens digestion. By following a glycemic index weight-loss program, however, you have a wonderful opportunity to pause and experience day-to-day eating in a different way. A more relaxing way. By now you've discovered the following things about glycemic index weight loss:

◆ You need to put more thought into your meals and snacks and actually plan them. You can't just grab something.

◆ It takes more time to chew vegetables and meats than to inhale a burger and fries. Plus, you know how quickly a person can eat a donut or cookie and still crave more.

◆ Even snacks need planning, because the snack machine at the office offers virtually nothing that is acceptable on a glycemic index meal plan.

◆ Many convenient snacks are still junk food and often high glycemic with more carbs than you can afford. Even some low-carb snack foods aren't consistent with the spirit of eating based on the glycemic index.

To say the least, your eating habits are already changing to support you staying at your ideal size for life. The following sections offer suggestions for making mealtimes more sensuous and pleasurable.

Lower the Stress Level

Eating when you're stressed isn't fun, and it's not great for your body. When your stress level is high, your body is in flight or fight mode. Your parasympathetic nervous system, which controls digestion, shuts down. When this happens, you're likely to experience indigestion or stomach discomfort. When stressed, your pleasure-sensing abilities diminish. You'll enjoy your meals much more if you decompress and de-stress before you take that first bite. Here are some suggestions for de-stressing before meals:

◆ Stretch or do some light movement, such as taking a walk

◆ Listen to music you love and sing along

◆ Have a cup of herbal or decaffeinated tea

◆ Chat with family and friends

◆ Say grace

Create some emotional and physical distance between your eating and other matters of your life. That way, when you do sit down to eat, you'll be able to focus on your food and give it your full attention.

Set the Atmosphere

Do you think of your eating environments as having an atmosphere in the same way that a restaurant owner knows that atmosphere can make or break a restaurant's success, regardless of how good the food is? Are you planning your eating scenario the same way a restaurant carefully plans its atmosphere?

Take a few moments to analyze your ideal eating environment and set it up for your weight-loss success. Follow these suggestions:

◆ Eat in a beautiful environment. Avoid eating at your desk or where you're working. Don't eat in your car. Instead, eat outside at a picnic table or at the dining room or kitchen table.

◆ Remove all clutter from the table and instead set the table with placemats, flatware, flowers, and candles to create a harmonious environment.

◆ Remove all clutter from your line of sight. That means dirty pots and pans, paperwork, and lists of chores to complete.

◆ Don't eat in front of the television. Turn it off. If you really want to watch a show, tape it and view it later.

◆ Listen to pleasant music or engage in uplifting conversation.

◆ Put your food on your plate before you bring it to the table. Don't put serving dishes on the table; you could be tempted to overeat.

◆ Before you sit down at the table, take a few moments to clear your mind from concerns and problems. Take a couple of deep breaths to release stress.

◆ Avoid discussing challenging or stressful topics while eating.

◆ If someone at the table misbehaves or is unpleasant, put down your fork and wait until the situation improves. Try not to get involved in the situation yourself.

Wrong Weigh

If you use eating as a way to soothe stress, it's time to make a change. Find a substitute activity such as exercise, reading, walking, or a hobby. Get to the root of your stressful feelings and make the necessary personal or lifestyle changes.

If you're feeling stressed, it's not the time to eat, it's time to relax. Learn more about managing stress on a glycemic index weight-loss program in Chapter 23.

Eat Slowly

Eating slowly is a good strategy for glycemic index weight loss. It will even help you keep your weight off. Ideally, a meal should take a minimum of 15 to 20 minutes—but preferably longer. Most of us eat way too fast. Slowing down offers many benefits:

Thin-spiration

Here's a way to learn to eat slowly. Ask a friend who you know eats really slowly to join you for lunch or dinner. Eat more slowly than your friend, even if you need to match her or him bite for bite. This may drive you crazy at first, but you'll learn how to slow down at meals.

- ◆ You have to be relaxed to eat slowly and to chew your food completely.

- ◆ You have more time to actually taste and enjoy your food.

- ◆ Your digestion improves.

- ◆ You can feel in your stomach when you've had enough to eat. When you eat quickly, it's more difficult to feel stomach satisfaction.

- ◆ Your food lasts longer so it seems as if you're eating more food, even though you aren't.

- ◆ You may not have time to eat all your food, in which case, either toss it out or store it for a snack later.

Slow eating is a reward in and of itself. You'll more than double your pleasure.

Reduce Distractions

Meals aren't pleasurable when you have lots of distractions. Not only are distractions annoying, they make it difficult to focus on enjoying your food. Here are some suggestions to eliminate distractions:

- ◆ Turn off the phone or don't answer it.

- ◆ Turn off the media—computers, cell phones, television, computer games, and radio (unless you are listening to background music).

- Don't answer the doorbell unless you expect company.
- Don't engage in arguments or disruptions with your children or other family members.

Thin-spiration

When you eat at a fine restaurant, you expect good service and no distractions. In fact, part of the price includes eating in a serene and beautiful environment. As best you can, create the same relaxing and calm ambience when you eat at home.

Wrong Weigh

Before you put that first bite of food into your mouth, sit down. Do this for every taste while you're cooking and for every morsel of food you want to eat when you're clearing the dishes. Sit to eat and you'll find that you won't be eating as much food as before.

Thin-spiration

The next time you go to a cocktail-type party, watch how people eat. People who are naturally thin aren't the people who stand near the stuffed mushrooms and pizza and eat continuously. They usually put food on a plate and then find a place to sit down and eat.

Depending on your family and their needs, reducing all distractions can be almost impossible. For example, babies can be fussy, and teenagers can be late to dinner. But within the realm of practicality, make your meals pleasant.

Eat Sitting Down

Stand-up eating was once considered impolite. But that was many years ago, before our nation was 67 percent overweight and expanding daily. Of course, sitting down to eat isn't necessarily healthier and it won't make you automatically thinner.

What sitting down does is let you relax and makes you aware that you're eating. Stand-up eating is often mindless, as when a person is snacking while cooking dinner or when standing in front of the sink looking out the kitchen window.

Be sure you don't eat standing up at a party, at the ball game, or at a backyard barbeque. Usually, when people eat while standing up, they eat faster and the foods they eat tend to be fast food or junk food. Seldom do people eat grilled salmon and salad when standing up. But they do eat chips, sodas, crackers, candy, and all the high-carb snack foods.

Three Meals a Day and More

One eating custom is virtually universal, practiced in nearly every culture around the world: eating three meals a day—breakfast, lunch, and dinner. This commonality suggests that we all need to eat at least three meals a day, because most people are hungry three times a day.

On the glycemic index weight-loss program, be sure to eat at least three times a day. Avoid skipping meals, because that can make your blood sugar levels and insulin levels unstable. Skipping meals also slows your metabolism—the very thing you don't want to happen.

Perhaps you've heard that snacking is bad for you. Not true. If you're hungry between meals, you can have a snack. Just make sure you include your snack in your total glycemic load intake for the day.

> **Thin-spiration**
>
> When Molly wanted a snack, she made sure she ate low-glycemic foods, but she wasn't gaining any sustenance from the snack. Instead she was gaining weight. Her typical snack consisted of a caffeinated diet soda and three or four artificially sweetened gelatin desserts. There wasn't any food in her snack. The caffeine triggered a rise in blood sugar levels resulting in a rise in insulin levels. Eating that much artificial sweetener was also inhibiting her weight loss, and even causing her to gain weight.
>
> Start getting in the habit now of eating foods that aren't as sweet-tasting.

Eat snacks that are nutritionally balanced. For example, half an avocado with salad dressing, a handful of nuts and an ounce of hard cheese, a hard boiled egg with a teaspoon of real mayonnaise, or a turkey and cheese roll-up. Eat regular food that's low in carbohydrates and high in nutrition.

Late-Night Eating

Late-night eating is in a whole different category than snacking. Usually raiding the refrigerator at night won't help your weight-loss program. Most late-night eating is …

♦ Mindless, meaning it's unplanned and not factored into a person's daily glycemic index eating program.

♦ Emotional eating. We've never heard of anyone who favors taking broiled fish filets to bed for a midnight snack. Instead, they choose high-starch, high-sugar, and high-carbohydrate comfort foods.

Avoid late-night eating. If you want a snack before bed, that's fine, but after you get into bed, don't eat until morning unless you have a doctor's instructions to do so.

The Least You Need to Know

- ◆ Use simple stress-reduction techniques to decompress before you start eating.
- ◆ Create an eating environment that's appealing, calm, and relaxing.
- ◆ Eat three meals a day plus snacks.
- ◆ Eat slowly and sit while eating.

Chapter **18**

Eating Out

In This Chapter

- ◆ Ordering at a restaurant
- ◆ Eating low-glycemic fast foods
- ◆ Dining at friends' homes
- ◆ Understanding low-carb restaurant menus

Eating out on a glycemic index weight-loss program is easier than you probably think. The rumors that it's hard were once true, but no longer. You know what to eat on a glycemic index weight-loss program, and now some of the people who plan restaurant menus are also clued in.

They want you to eat out and they want you to eat out often. Sure, you may need to forego some special whole-grain breads and other unique low-glycemic treats, but eating out, dining out, going through the drive-through, or eating at the buffet has never been easier.

This chapter guides you through the process of ordering meals at restaurants. You learn how and what to order and how to negotiate with the waitperson. You also learn how to eat at friends' homes and stay true to your glycemic index way of eating.

Restaurants

The fundamental ingredients of glycemic index eating are the basic foods that make up most restaurant meals. Meats, fish, poultry, vegetables, and fruit are all-time standards. Provided that a restaurant offers those basics, they can serve you food to meet your weight-loss needs.

If you view glycemic index eating this way, you can be comfortable ordering a meal in virtually any restaurant. You don't need to be intimidated—remember, the restaurant is there to meet your needs. Not the other way around.

Wrong Weigh

Finding balanced, low-glycemic meals can be challenging at two types of restaurants. The first is at vegetarian restaurants, especially if they don't serve any animal proteins, such as meat or fish. The second is, surprisingly, salad bars. Often, salad bars skimp on their offerings of animal protein and instead offer bits of meat or fish in pasta salads and serve up shredded hard cheeses. If you can find a salad bar where you can eat three ounces of high-quality animal protein at a meal, then go ahead and eat there. If not, pass on these types of restaurants.

Ordering from the Menu

Let's make ordering as easy as possible. For lunches and dinners, start with an entrée. Bypass the pastas and pizzas, and let your eyes cruise through the salads, entrées, and sandwiches.

Yes, we said sandwiches. Sandwiches can offer delicious combinations of meats and cheeses. However, it's highly unlikely that a sandwich shop will have low-glycemic bread. When you order a sandwich, just ask the server to hold the bread. They know how to do this. Also ask whether you can substitute a small salad for the French fries or chips.

Select the main-dish salad or entrée that sounds the best. Be sure to ask the server to hold the bread and croutons. If you want an appetizer, order one that contains vegetables and meats and skip the ones with high amounts of starches, such as quesadillas, cornbread, or those that are bread-based.

Tossed salads and main-dish salads always work for glycemic index weight-loss, as do sautéed or steamed vegetables. If you want the artichoke cheese dip as an appetizer, be sure to ask the server to bring some cut vegetables instead of crackers or bread for dipping.

Desserts can really be tempting. At this point you need to select your discretionary foods. Most of the time, you won't have any left for the day. But if you do, you can order dessert provided that you …

◆ Don't eat it all.

◆ Have confidence that you can take the rest home and eat a bite a day until it's gone.

◆ Have three or four people at the table each eat a bite or two.

A taste can be just as powerful to your taste buds as a portion. And you'll definitely like the long-term results more.

Don't Super-Size

Super-sized meals are way too big for you. They contain more food than you need. Don't order them. Instead, half-size your meals by sharing your entrée with a friend.

Most restaurant portions are huge—big enough for two and sometimes even large enough for three people. That is, unless you are eating at a very fine—meaning expensive—restaurant. Only then do the portion sizes relate in any way to the size of your stomach.

You can stretch your "eat-out" budget while eating a right-sized meal. Share the entrée and meal with a friend. Restaurant servers are great at handling this situation. Often, they split the entrées and side salads in the kitchen. If they don't, ask for an extra plate.

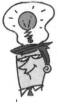

Thin-spiration

You don't need to explain to the server that you are eating based on the glycemic index unless you want to. Sometimes it might seem helpful, but as you gather experience and confidence, ordering will become second nature to you.

Thin-spiration

When in doubt about what to order, think animal proteins, such as meat, seafood, or poultry and vegetables. Fill at least half of your plate with vegetables, the rest with animal proteins and then add another side dish of salad, vegetables, or fruit.

Thin-spiration

Suzi and Jack always share an entrée when they eat out at restaurants, and even sometimes at fast-food places. They say they each get plenty to eat and that often they end up taking some food home—usually enough for one person's lunch the next day. They spend less and actually enjoy leaving the table feeling comfortable and not stuffed.

At the Buffet

You may find it trickier to navigate your way through a buffet line than at a "sit-down and be served" restaurant. Too many choices, too much food, and often, but not always, way too many high-glycemic choices.

There are exceptions. Some Sunday buffet brunches are often simply wonderful. They offer vegetables, salads, eggs, and meats. When they are truly elaborate, you can eat seafood, Eggs Benedict (hold the muffin), and delightful fruit. Your challenge is to only put the foods on your plate that look most appealing and to be highly discerning about the foods you don't want to eat.

But most buffets are more challenging. Here's how to approach the buffet line. Go backward. Survey the line starting at the end, where the good stuff is, such as prime rib and salmon. Then walk toward the front of the line, planning which foods to put on your plate. Remember, your tummy has a limited amount of room. Following are tips for getting through the line:

♦ On your first pass, avoid filling up your plate with foods placed at the start of the line. Instead, save room on your plate for the best foods placed toward the end of the line. Take the plate back to your seat and eat slowly and sensuously. Remember, at the buffet there is always plenty of food.

Thin-spiration

Believe it or not, it's totally possible to develop a dislike for doughy, sweet foods and sweetened beverages. Many people have done this. By now you know they make you feel bloated, may give you gas, wheezing, or a runny nose. Plus, that doughy feeling in your mouth can get disgusting.

♦ If and only if you have more room in your stomach, take a second walk through the line, taking morsels and bites or even seconds of some of your favorites.

♦ Make the pastries, cereals, and breads invisible. Train yourself not to see them until you develop a true dislike for them. They're what other people eat, not what you eat.

♦ If there's any room left in your stomach, ask for a bite of a friend's dessert. Or just order tea or coffee and finish your meal with a light feeling in your stomach.

Use this same technique for buffets at holiday parties and summer picnics. Just because it's on the table doesn't mean it needs to be in your mouth or stomach. Now that many people are also eating based on the glycemic index, you may find yourself delighted with the offerings at potluck dinners and tailgate parties.

Fast Food

They're everywhere—on virtually every city street corner and at stops along the highway. They're convenient. They offer inexpensive food. So what's the problem?

The most popular menu offerings at fast-food restaurants are high-glycemic, high in carbohydrates, and high in high-fructose corn syrup. They offer all the eating components you want to avoid. But—and here's the good news—things are changing in the fast-food world, and they're changing fast.

Fast-food restaurants want to meet your needs—they want your business—so they now offer menu choices based on the glycemic index. Here are some suggestions for eating fast food that's low in carbohydrates:

- Order a hamburger or cheeseburger (hold the bun) with a small salad. Ask for a glass of water.

- Never "super-size" anything.

- If everyone else wants pizza, go ahead and order it with a salad. Eat the salad. You can also have a slice or two of pizza, but eat your pizza differently. Peel off the topping and eat it. Toss out the crust. You are able to eat the best part of the pizza and savor the taste.

- Order a submarine sandwich in either a wrap or bread. Also ask for a fork and knife. Ask to have your sandwich prepared with all the salad toppings. Open up the sandwich or wrap and eat the insides with fork and knife. If the shop will hold the bread, ask them to do that.

Wrong Weigh

Just because you're eating fast food doesn't mean you need to eat fast. Instead, eat slowly, eat sitting down, and eat in as pleasant an environment as possible. Don't eat while driving.

Thin-spiration

Some of the low-carb wraps offered at sandwich shops are high in fiber and also low-glycemic. If a low-carb wrapping fits into your allotted glycemic load for that meal, then eat the wrap along with the vegetables, meats, and cheeses inside.

Wrong Weigh

Substituting a wrap for sandwich bread may not save you very many carbohydrates. Check the carb listing before you take a bite. Ask yourself whether you really want to use up your carb grams for the day on bread.

◆ Order the main-dish salad, which can be quite delicious and low in carbohydrates. Use some of the salad dressing. You might want to pass on the croutons, crunchy noodles, sugared almonds, and sweetened oranges. Usually, the salad by itself is low-glycemic, but the added condiments are usually high-glycemic.

◆ We haven't seen any beverage offerings that are completely suitable for a glycemic index weight-loss program. They are either full of high-fructose corn syrup, aspartame, and/or caffeine. Even an 8-ounce glass of juice has too high a glycemic load. Your best beverage choice as of this writing is plain water or herbal tea.

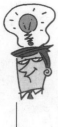

Thin-spiration

Wouldn't it be great to be able to order a cup of herbal tea at a fast-food restaurant? Until that day, take a tea bag with you and order a cup of hot water.

◆ Fried chicken works if you remove the skin before you eat it. Eat the coleslaw by draining off some of the sugary liquid. Pass on the biscuits and mashed potatoes. Absolutely pass on the honey blend; it contains less honey and more high-glycemic sugar syrups.

◆ Eat the fillings of tacos and burritos with a fork and pass on the tortillas. Ditto with taco salads.

As you eat at fast-food restaurants, you're going to find more menu choices based on the glycemic index. Be sure to read the fine print before you indulge. Remember, you can't go wrong with a burger (hold the bun) and a salad.

At a Friend's Home

Eating based on the glycemic index at a friend's home is tricky. Perhaps you've had people over for dinner and noticed that one person wasn't eating. You find out too late that the person is allergic to the foods you offered or was for some other reason unable to eat them. Gosh, how you wish that person had phoned you ahead of time and discussed his or her dietary needs. It would have saved both of you the discomfort of embarrassment.

Here are some suggestions for eating based on the glycemic index at a friend's home:

◆ Call ahead and ask whether you can bring a dish or beverage. That way, you can bring foods or beverages that fit into your glycemic index eating program.

◆ Call ahead at least a week in advance and tell your host or hostess that you're on a glycemic index weight-loss program and have some dietary restrictions. You can ask what the menu is. If the planned menu won't work at all for you, offer to bring a side dish that will.

◆ If your host or hostess asks whether you have any food preferences, keep your answer simple. Basically, you can eat meat, fish, and vegetables. So say that and avoid elaborate requests. You want to be invited back, and getting food-fussy at a party isn't fun for anyone.

◆ If worse comes to worst, you can pick at your food, claim not to be hungry, and then eat later on the way home or at home. Of course, this isn't ideal, but it might be necessary.

> **Wrong Weigh**
>
> Allison went to a wedding reception totally unprepared. Every dish of food was filled with breads or sweets. Even the tuna-fish sandwiches were unacceptable on her glycemic index weight-loss program. They were fluffy croissants each filled with about a teaspoon of salad. The salads were Jell-O–based. All the beverages were sugary. She made it through the party by eating a few raw vegetables and later stopped on the way home for an acceptable meal. Had she known, she could have packed a couple of hard-boiled eggs in her handbag.

Eating meals at a friend's home isn't really about the food, it's about the friendship and good times. Don't let the food get in the way. Eat ahead, eat at the party, eat after the party, but make the most of your friendships. They'll last long after you've attained your ideal size.

Take-Along Food

Now that you're eating very differently, don't get caught without food when you need it. Perhaps you decided to head out shopping at about 3 P.M. After an hour, you're starving. You need food and you need it now. What are you going to do?

It's really easy to find unacceptable foods at malls and shopping areas. But you don't want to eat candy, sugary beverages, or cookies. Let's face it—food vendors at the malls don't sell hard-boiled eggs, carrot sticks, or raw fruit.

This is the time when you need to be your own best friend. Never leave home without some kinds of acceptable foods. Keep these foods in your glove compartment, handbag, backpack, or briefcase. You can also keep them in your desk at work. Acceptable snacks include the following:

♦ Small containers of hard cheese that don't require refrigeration.

♦ Small containers of peanut butter that don't require refrigeration.

♦ Nuts, such as pecans, peanuts, hazelnuts, cashews, and almonds.

♦ Dried apricots, because they're low glycemic, as are dried pears, peaches, and apples. Eat only a couple.

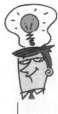

> **Thin-spiration**
>
> Use an insulated container to carry foods with more variety. That way you can carry salads with cottage cheese, poultry, and meat.

> **Body of Knowledge**
>
> You may have read or heard that carrots are high-glycemic, but they are, in fact, low. Early testing methods found them to be high, but it simply wasn't reasonable that the only high-glycemic vegetable was carrots. Recent tests show them to be low, whether cooked or raw.

♦ Small cans of tuna or sardines. Pack along a plastic fork and paper napkin.

♦ Beef or buffalo jerky, preferably homemade or made without preservatives and artificial coloring.

♦ Raw carrots, celery, radishes, and other raw vegetables.

♦ Water. If you are in your car frequently, keep a one-gallon container of purified water and some water bottles in your car. Often a glass of water can ease hunger for a half hour until you can find a place to eat.

♦ Black or green olives in a waterproof container.

♦ Coarsely ground low-glycemic whole-grain products such as crackers and bread. You can also add some al dente whole-grain pasta to your salads.

By packing these kinds of food items and eating them when you get hungry, you can avoid becoming so hungry that you want to eat a horse—that is, a horse made of sugar and dough.

Low-Carb Restaurant Foods

Many restaurants offer low-carb entrées and appetizers. This sounds great, and certainly the restaurants want to meet your needs. But take care and read the fine print.

Sometimes you're going to be better off ordering a steak and salad than choosing a low-carb food.

Here's how to check out the low-carb menu:

◆ Ask to see the ingredient list. If the chef won't show you the list or claims to add secret ingredients to the recipe, don't order the food. Food labels at the grocery store need to have full disclosure of ingredients, and there's no good reason why a chef should keep his ingredients secret from you. After all, you're the person who's doing the eating.

◆ Be sure that the carbohydrate count is accurate for the portion you're served. Sometimes the carb count is for half or one third the serving size.

◆ Beware of low-carb breads, muffins, tortillas, and chips. To produce a low-carb bread-type product, the baker needs to use some odd ingredients, and you want to know what they are before you order. Plus they may be high-glycemic.

◆ Ask whether the food is also low-glycemic. Some low-carb foods are high-glycemic, so the glycemic load could be higher than you want to eat.

◆ Ask whether the food is artificially sweetened. If so, pass on it.

Wrong Weigh

Low-carb foods and menus aren't the same as low-glycemic. A food can be low in total carbohydrate count, and still be high in glycemic index or glycemic load. Don't be fooled into thinking that by eating a low-carb entrée you're eating based on the glycemic index.

Weeding out healthful food offerings from those with more marketing hype than substance is challenging to anyone who wants to eat based on the glycemic index. Fortunately, you already know the basics: animal proteins and vegetables. You can eat out well forever without ever partaking of a restaurant's low-carbohydrate processed food. When you find a low-carb offering that's also good for you, enjoy.

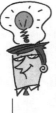

Thin-spiration

In an ideal world, all restaurants would list the glycemic load per serving, along with net carbs and glycemic index. Then you would know exactly how the food will affect your blood sugar levels, as well as whether it will increase insulin resistance. We can only hope that inspired food manufacturers will eventually give us this information.

The Least You Need to Know

 ◆ You can always eat low-glycemic by ordering animal proteins and vegetables—
   hold the breads and desserts.

 ◆ Don't be intimidated by restaurant servers—their job is to serve you the foods
   that you want to eat.

 ◆ Fast-food restaurants now offer main-dish salads and side salads that work for
   the glycemic index weight loss program.

 ◆ Carry low-glycemic snacks with you so that you never need to resort to eating
   unacceptable foods when hungry.

Chapter 19

Shopping Based on the Glycemic Index

In This Chapter

- ◆ Selecting grocery store foods
- ◆ Buying meats and vegetables
- ◆ Selecting packaged foods
- ◆ Frequenting your health-food store

You've spent years knowing exactly how to shop for groceries. You may have even memorized what to purchase from each aisle, and you certainly know how to shop the specials. So, who would have thought you would ever need to relearn such a basic skill as grocery shopping?

If you've followed any of the advice in this book so far, your shopping habits are already changing. You're reading product ingredient lists and may be amazed at how many processed and high-glycemic carbohydrates are found in seemingly innocent foods. Little did you realize just how many carbs you once ate on a daily basis.

In this chapter, you learn guidelines for how to shop for glycemic index weight loss and for weight maintenance. You'll find the new way of shopping just as easy as before, and you'll find new foods and be able to experience new culinary delights.

At the Grocery Store

As you review your weekly grocery shopping list, here's what you're going to find. Most of the foods on your list are available at the outside perimeter of the store, in the frozen-food section, or in the health-food section. In fact, with the exception of condiments, spices, olive oil, and vinegar, you never need to walk down the food aisles packed full with carbohydrate-rich foods.

It's possible that you won't find some of the items on your list at the grocery store at all, in which case you should visit a health-food store once or twice a month. How to shop at health-food stores is discussed later in this chapter. The following sections discuss how to shop at the grocery store.

Body of Knowledge

Today, the fat in beef is more unsaturated than it was 10 years ago. Many cattle are now both range-fed and grain-fed, which results in less saturated fat in the meat. Ten years ago, most cattle were only grain-fed.

Thin-spiration

Always keep a few pounds of lean ground beef in your freezer. With a pound of ground beef you can make hamburgers, taco mix for Mexican main courses, or Italian meat sauce to serve with spaghetti squash or a half cup of whole-wheat al dente pasta. You can even serve it over cooked cauliflower—believe it or not, it tastes great.

Shopping for Animal Protein

You have many choices for animal protein that give you great taste and can also be easy on your budget.

- **Beef.** This food is a reliable pleaser and is highly versatile for your glycemic index weight-loss program. Your choices include cuts that cook up quickly on the grill, such as lean ground beef and steaks, roasts for the oven or slow-cooker, precut strips for sautéing, and flank steak to marinate and cook on the grill or in the oven.

Don't forget sliced roast beef, ham, or turkey from the deli counter to eat for breakfast or lunchtime roll-ups and as late-afternoon snacks. You can even serve them warmed up with eggs for breakfast.

- **Pork.** Pork adds variety and many pork cuts are low in fat, such as pork chops, tenderloin, ham, and roasts. Pork ribs are excellent—slow-cook to render off the fat, and then crisp up in the oven or on the grill. Pork sausage tends to be very fatty, so you may want to pass on it and select turkey sausage instead. But be sure to check the labels, because some turkey sausage is also quite high in fat. By trimming off excess fat, you can more easily keep your daily fat intake at 30 percent of your food.

◆ **Chicken and turkey.** Poultry readily picks up the flavors of other foods, such as condiments, spices, and any vegetables it's cooked with. Grocery stores offer a wide variety of prepackaged choices: drumsticks, breasts, strips for fajitas, and breast pieces for stews and quick sautéing. Purchase whole turkeys or just the turkey breast for roasting. You'll have meat left over for cold cuts and for snacks.

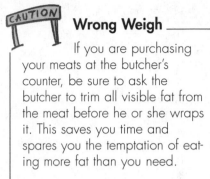

Wrong Weigh

If you are purchasing your meats at the butcher's counter, be sure to ask the butcher to trim all visible fat from the meat before he or she wraps it. This saves you time and spares you the temptation of eating more fat than you need.

◆ **Specialty meats.** Don't forget to consider cooking with lamb, veal, and Cornish game hens. Many people favor buffalo and game, such as duck, pheasant, and elk. You can find many excellent low-glycemic recipes for specialty meats.

◆ **Seafood.** Shellfish and fish taste best when purchased fresh and eaten within a day. You can also freeze them, if you need to. Avoid purchasing seafood that's already been frozen and then thawed. You need to eat it right away, and you can't refreeze it. If you can't find fresh-caught fish, purchase it frozen and store it in your freezer until you're ready to thaw and cook it.

◆ **Eggs.** Plan to always keep eggs on hand. Sauté some for breakfast or hard-boil them for brown-bag lunches and tuna or salmon salads. Eggs stay fresh for weeks in your refrigerator.

◆ **Canned and prepackaged fish and meats.** Think tuna, salmon, and sardines. These are available in cans and prepackaged in plastic and foil bags. Keep some on hand for traveling, snacks, and quick lunches or breakfasts. Canned salmon and tuna are usually caught wild.

◆ **Bacon.** A few slices a couple of times a month is a treat. Bacon only contains about two grams of protein per slice, so you need to add other protein to your meal to eat the recommended 15 to 20 grams of animal protein per meal. Purchase the kind of bacon you like best. Because bacon is very high in saturated fat, use it sparingly. Be sure to pour off the fat before you serve it and toss out the rendered fat. You can also purchase turkey bacon or pork bacon. Be sure to read the fat content on the label to make sure the turkey bacon is indeed lower in fat.

Thin-spiration

For an unusually tasty treat, occasionally (once a month) you can purchase thinly sliced salami. To cook, spread on paper towels on a microwavable plate. Microwave on high for 30 seconds or until the salami is crisp. It's great for snacks and also good crumbled up in salads. One slice or two is very satisfying. And, good news, most of the fat is absorbed by the paper towels.

At the Deli

Consider the deli to be your quick-meal resource center. You can purchase whole roasted chickens and a wide variety of sliced meats and cheeses. You may want to pass on the salads because they tend to be high in processed carbohydrates. Definitely avoid salads made with white pastas, grains, and flavored gelatin. Instead, look for tossed vegetable salads and coleslaws, provided they aren't drenched in sugar and salad dressing. Whole roasted chicken is often available and a good choice. Fried chicken is high in trans-fatty acids.

Vegetables

So many vegetables, so little time. If you're like most people in the vegetable section of the grocery store, you buy the same vegetables over and over again and never even think to try something new. Now is the time to shop this section with new eyes.

You'll find snow peapods, fennel root, celery root, and spaghetti squash. And that's just a start. Now that you are eating 5 to 10 servings of vegetables and fruits a day, increase your variety. Cooking directions are usually on the labels, and if not, ask the produce experts at the store. Here are some tips about purchasing vegetables:

- ◆ Purchase fresh or frozen. Fresh vegetables keep about a week in the vegetable crisper of your refrigerator. Frozen keep much longer. Keep frozen vegetables as a backup in case you run out of fresh produce during the week.

- ◆ Frozen vegetables are a great choice because they are frozen at optimal ripeness. Fresh produce is often harvested weeks before it arrives at the grocer's shelves and may have lost important nutrients in transit.

- ◆ Prepackaged lettuces and vegetables that are cleaned and cut are convenient, but perhaps cost more. The baby carrots and trimmed romaine hearts may be worth it. If you want convenience, shop the prepackaged sections.

- ◆ Use spices and condiments to jazz up vegetables. Try a sprinkle of dried tarragon on cauliflower, curry on broccoli, and cilantro on tomatoes. The spices and herbs bring out the flavor of vegetables. Eat them plain, or eat them spiced, but be sure to eat them.

◆ Purchase or grow fresh herbs to add to salads. Chopped fresh basil, tarragon, parsley, cilantro, and others add zest and interest to a tossed green salad. You can find sun-dried tomatoes in the produce section. Add a mere teaspoon in sauces, meat, or over vegetables to give them a delicious Mediterranean flavor.

Vegetables give your mouth and stomach satisfaction. Eaten raw, they're crunchy and have plenty of fiber. Cook your vegetables to the al dente stage, meaning still a bit crunchy, so that you enjoy the mouth satisfaction that vegetables offer.

In the summer and fall, you can shop for vegetables and fruit at local farmers' markets. These seem to be sprouting up in many locations all over the country. Usually, the produce is locally grown and picked fresh. Take cash, because you may not be able to pay with a credit card. Going to a farmers' market allows you to support local growers and get fresh produce weekly.

Fruit

Fruit is nature's candy. It tastes sweet, satisfies your sweet tooth, and is full of important nutrients and antioxidants. Plus, most fruit is low-glycemic.

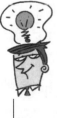

Thin-spiration

In many parts of the country, it's hard to purchase fresh berries that are ripe and in good shape without being moldy. If you live in one of those areas, try frozen berries. Find them unsweetened in resealable plastic bags in the freezer section of the grocery store. They're yummy and delicious eaten plain or in a glass parfait with whipped low-fat cream cheese. Plus, berries are low-glycemic.

Choose more common fruits, such as apples and pears, or shop for more exotic fare, such as pomegranates and papayas. When eating, savor the natural sweetness, texture, and juiciness of the fruit.

Cheese

Your grocery store offers a great selection of common cheeses from around the world. Your health-food store and natural-food grocers may have some more exotic varieties.

Choose your favorite hard or soft cheeses, such as cheddar, Brie, cream cheese, and Parmesan. In a sense, the world's the limit on what cheeses you eat. Both low-fat and regular cheeses are low-glycemic. However, use both in moderation.

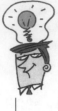

Thin-spiration

Shredded and grated Parmesan cheese is almost mandatory as a kitchen staple, right up there with salt and pepper. Add a bit of shredded Parmesan to eggs, salads, and cooked vegetables. Add it to cottage cheese and sprinkle over spaghetti sauce. It's salty and tangy, so just a little bit will go far in enhancing flavor, and it is lower in fat than many of the regular full-fatted cheeses.

Whole Grains and Cereals

Get ready to read the list of ingredients. Here's what to look for:

- **Brown rice.** This rice is already a whole grain and it has more fiber and more nutrients than white rice. Wild rice is a good choice and is a whole grass, not a grain, but you cook and serve it just as you would regular rice. When you purchase rice, check out the glycemic index of that variety of rice. The glycemic indexes of rice range from low to high.

- **Whole-grain pasta.** The whole-grain variety is now available in most grocery stores. Remember to cook it al dente for low-glycemic eating.

- **Corn tortillas and whole-wheat tortillas.** Corn tortillas are medium-, while whole-wheat tortillas are high-glycemic. Low-carb whole-wheat tortillas are lower-glycemic than the regular whole-wheat tortillas, plus they have a lower-glycemic load.

- **Breads.** If you can find true coarsely ground whole-grain bread, buy it. But most store-bought breads contain enriched or white flour, as well as sugars and some mystery ingredients. If the bread, muffin, hard roll, or hamburger bun isn't made with 100 percent whole-wheat flour, pass on it. Some specialty bread shops offer truly whole-grain breads. While most whole-wheat and white-wheat breads are high-glycemic, authentic stone-ground breads are medium.

- **Cookies, cakes, and other baked goods.** It's unlikely that any of these products are totally whole grain. Most cookies and cakes are medium-glycemic because they're made with

Wrong Weigh

Caramel coloring is often added to breads and bread products to make them appear to contain more whole wheat than they do. Don't buy them and instead look for bread that is truly 100 percent whole grain.

butter or oil, which lowers the glycemic index value. Whole grain is great, but you can eat small amounts of cookies and cake and still lose weight provided that your glycemic load stays in range for the meal and the day.

- ◆ **Cereals.** With the exception of All-Bran, Muesli, some Kashi cereals, and steel-cut oats, breakfast cereals are high- or medium-glycemic and are often filled with refined or enriched flours and grains. You may want to eat animal protein, vegetables, and fruit for breakfast and only occasionally eat breakfast cereals. The fluffier the cereal, the higher-glycemic. Added sugar makes it even higher-glycemic.

- ◆ **Other grains.** Barley, wheat berries, rye kernels, cracked wheat, and buckwheat groats are grains you may enjoy. If you can't find them at the grocery store, you can purchase them at health-food stores. These grains are low-glycemic products.

When selecting and eating grains and cereals, be sure you don't fall back into the eating rut you were in before you began your glycemic index weight-loss program. Eat them sparingly, still focusing on making animal protein and vegetables the mainstay of your meals and snacks.

Dairy, Nuts, and Other Foods

Always select low-fat or nonfat dairy products (other than regular cheese) to keep your fat intake lower. Milk and plain yogurt are low-glycemic but have plenty of carbohydrates, so eat or drink them with wisdom and care.

Many grocers now offer larger packages of nuts in the produce section. Overall, they're a better buy than the small packages of nuts near the baking supplies and spices. Use nuts for snacks and salad toppings in moderation. Pickles, capers, vinegars, anchovies, and other condiments make good recipes even better. As these are generally low-glycemic (one exception is sweet pickles), have fun with your shopping.

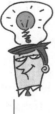

Thin-spiration

Stock up on acidic condiments, such as dill pickles, capers, mustard, chutney, onions, vinegars, sauerkraut, horseradish, and marinated vegetables such as mushrooms and artichoke hearts. Choose tangy salsas made without added sugars and select bottles of authentic lemon or lime juice. Eat these with your meals to naturally lower the glycemic load of the meal.

Oils and Butter

If you could only purchase one of these, you would want to keep olive oil in your kitchen. This is all you need for dressing salads and cooking. If you want more varieties of oils, be sure to purchase only cold-expeller pressed vegetable or nut oils, such as walnut oil or canola oil. You'll probably find wider selections at health-food stores.

Avoid purchasing margarines and fake butters that are made with partially hydrogenated vegetable oils. Those are the same as trans-fatty acids, and they don't belong in anyone's stomach because they can cause heart disease.

Use monounsaturated oils such as canola oil for sautéing and cooking, and olive oil for dressing salads and vegetables. You can use butter, but it's best to use it in small amounts so that you keep your saturated fat intake to under 10 percent of your food consumption. A small amount is one teaspoon a couple of times a week.

Shopping the Low-Carb Aisle

Most grocery stores now have a low-carb aisle that offers prepackaged low-carb foods. In truth, many of the foods in grocery stores, such as meats and vegetables, are already low in carbohydrates and low-glycemic. And some of them are quite convenient.

So what's in the low-carb aisle? Mostly snack foods and baked-good mixes. You'll find some condiments, such as catsup, made without sugar, but perhaps made with artificial sweeteners. Low-carb foods can be high-glycemic, so be very selective. Also, some of these products have unnecessarily high amounts of saturated and trans-fats.

If you want to shop this aisle, you need to read labels and ingredient lists. The foods may or may not be supportive of your eating plan. For example, if the food contains artificial sweeteners, white or enriched flours, high fat, maltodextrins, or modified food starches, you won't benefit from eating it.

Some of the foods are good for you, such as some whole-wheat tortillas and some baked goods. Perhaps you look forward to the day when all foods at the grocery store offer you optimal nutrition and wholesome eating. We do, too.

Wrong Weigh

Just because a food is marketed as being low in carbohydrates doesn't mean that you can eat it indiscriminately—it may not be low-glycemic. If the food meets your criteria for a wholesome food, then eat it in moderation, being sure not to overeat. Remember that overeating all by itself can cause insulin resistance and weight gain.

At the Health-Food Store

If you haven't already, it's time to get to know your local health-food store. Not just the part of the store with shelves filled with vitamins and supplements, but the natural-foods section that offers natural foods, cheeses, bulk nuts, and legumes.

Put these foods on your health-food store shopping list:

- Bulk psyllium for proper elimination and to add fiber to your diet. Psyllium is a grain with no carbs that provides fiber. Psyllium isn't listed on the glycemic index list because it has no net carbohydrates. To use, add 1 tablespoon psyllium to a large glass of water and drink immediately. Follow up with a smaller glass of water.

- Bulk flaxseeds. To obtain the highest nutritional benefit, grind the flaxseeds before eating. Flaxseeds can be ground in a small coffee grinder at home. After grinding, store in the freezer to protect the valuable omega-3 fatty acids from becoming rancid. Sprinkle on salads, eggs, and vegetables. Don't use for cooking or baking as heat can damage the value of the essential fatty acid content.

- Whole grains. These often come in bulk. Use for pilafs and side dishes.

- Steel-cut oats (also called thick-cut oats in some stores). Make hot cereal with these oats. The cooking time is about 20 to 30 minutes.

- Wild rice. It often costs less at health-food stores.

- Dried apricots, pears, and peaches in bulk. These are low-glycemic and good for snacks during your maintenance phase.

- Organic milk, yogurt, and butter. If you want to eat organic, try these.

- Specialty cheeses.

- Nuts in bulk.

Health-food stores may have better prices than grocery stores. If you want to eat organic, you can shop for meats and vegetables here as well. Read the grocery store and health-food store promotional fliers every week so you can take advantage of meat and fish specials, as well as specials on frozen vegetables and fruit.

The Least You Need to Know

◆ You need to develop new grocery-shopping habits for your glycemic index weight-loss program.

◆ Purchase most foods around the perimeter of the grocery store and only some in the aisles.

◆ Select either fresh or frozen vegetables and fruits.

◆ Shop at a health-food market for whole grains and some bulk items, such as nuts and seeds.

Chapter 20

Cooking Based on the Glycemic Index

In This Chapter

- ◆ Starting with animal proteins and vegetables
- ◆ Using recipes and cookbooks
- ◆ Cooking for yourself or a family
- ◆ Packing meals and snacks

Now that you're cooking based on the glycemic index, you need a new answer to the question "What's for dinner?" Your answer might have once been "Meat and potatoes." Or perhaps it was "Takeout."

Your new answer is quite simple. "It will be healthy and wonderful!" The answer holds true whether you're eating takeout, cooking in, or planning a dinner party or outdoor barbeque.

Cooking based on the glycemic index might be new to you, but it's more balanced and healthy, and it's actually easier than many other ways of cooking. You'll be using animal protein (red meat, seafood, or poultry), small amounts of healthy fats, and lower-glycemic, unprocessed carbohydrates including vegetables, fruit, some whole grains, nuts and seeds, some dairy, and spices and condiments. When these ingredients are properly prepared, you'll have the makings of a delicious and nutritious meal.

Gustatory Delights

Somehow the very thought of meat and vegetables sounds dry and stiff, which certainly isn't appetizing. But don't let the sound fool you. Glycemic index weight-loss meals can be stunning and either simple or complex to prepare—based on your preference.

We've served glycemic index weight-loss meals to guests who have battled over licking the last drops of sauce from the bowl of a simple dish called Fennel and Tomatoes. Dinner guests have eaten every last bite of Paprika Chicken, as well as Pork Chops with Raisins and Walnuts. Try the Basil Pot Roast—you'll love it. You can find these and other recipes based on the glycemic index in *The Complete Idiot's Guide to Low-Carb Meals* and *The Complete Idiot's Guide to Terrific Diabetic Meals.*

Thin-spiration

You can find glycemic-index cooking classes at kitchen stores and diabetic teaching centers. Call and ask for a schedule and attend some classes. You'll gather plenty of ideas you can use, plus you'll enjoy the eating.

It's easy for anyone to give up on a weight-loss program when the food is unfamiliar, odd, or extreme. Cooking for glycemic index weight loss is none of these things after you figure it out. In essence, all you're doing is substituting lower-glycemic foods (whole, unprocessed starches and sugars) for high-glycemic foods (those that are high in refined starches and sugars). Now's the time to figure it out.

Planning Meals

Whether you like to carefully preplan your weekly meals or prepare foods more spontaneously, the following glycemic index cooking basics will work well for you:

♦ About one fourth of each meal should be from an animal protein. Think eggs, meat, seafood, poultry, or cheese for breakfast, lunch, and dinner.

♦ Add in vegetables for all meals. Prepare two vegetables or two vegetable servings per meal. Make sure that vegetables comprise about half your meal.

♦ The final fourth of the meal should consist of yams, legumes, fruit, dairy, whole-grain pasta, or brown rice.

◆ If you need to keep your glycemic load low, use spaghetti squash to substitute for spaghetti, zucchini slices to substitute for lasagna noodles, and mashed, cooked cauliflower in place of mashed potatoes.

 Thin-spiration

If you're looking for a soothing hobby, consider gardening. That way, you can grow fresh vegetables and fruit such as lettuce, strawberries, carrots, and more. You can reap the culinary rewards of your efforts, plus enjoy a creative and relaxing hobby.

◆ You can use lettuce leaves to hold sandwich fillings, or use cabbage or slices of jicama instead of low-glycemic breads if you need to keep your glycemic load low.

◆ If you want dessert, bake or cook some recipes from the many excellent low-glycemic and low-carb cookbooks available. Be sure to avoid cooking with artificial sweeteners, because they can actually increase your appetite and could be harmful to your health. Instead, use stevia with FOS for sweetening.

◆ Get creative. Spread nut butters on slices of apples, peaches, or pears for an out-of-this-world delicious treat. Ditto on cheese. A serving size of nut butters is $1/2$ tablespoon.

◆ Always cook more meat for dinner than you and your family can eat. The leftovers are great for breakfast, lunch, the next night's dinner, and snacks. However, leftover fish is usually awful unless it's salmon or tuna. You can make tuna or salmon salad with the leftovers.

◆ Keep cut-up carrots and celery in the refrigerator. Eat them by themselves or add some nut butter or cheese for an instant snack. You can also keep slices of radishes, jicama, green and red peppers, broccoli, cauliflower, and so on (the list is almost endless) in the refrigerator.

Body of Knowledge

When planning meals for your maintenance program, remember that low-glycemic starches are only one fourth of the total volume of the meal. That's only one fourth of the space on your plate! For example, a couple of croutons on a salad and half of a small yam is about one fourth of the space on your plate. A few corn tortilla chips with guacamole salad is fine, but pass on the sopapillas (Mexican fried dessert bread made with white flour). Prepare your own croutons with sourdough bread cubes to lower the glycemic index of regular croutons.

- Clean lettuce once a week, when you are putting the groceries away, to avoid cleaning lettuce every time you prepare a salad. It'll keep for a week in the crisper.

- If you don't already have one, purchase a slow cooker. Then let meats such as pork ribs, chuck roast, and pork loin simmer during the day. At dinner, the meat's ready to eat and all you need to do is cook some vegetables and/or make a tossed salad for dinner.

- Use the outdoor grill as a quick way to cook meats, fish, and vegetables without needing to clean pots and pans after dinner.

- Keep condiments such as shredded Parmesan cheese, spices and herbs, olive oil, vinegar, sun-dried tomatoes, and garlic on hand.

- Because acidic foods lower the glycemic index, keep plenty of acidic condiments in your pantry and refrigerator and serve them with your meals.

- Clear out the foods you won't be eating any longer. Food banks welcome your contributions of canned goods and unopened prepackaged foods.

> **Body of Knowledge**
>
> Some cookbooks for persons with diabetes are based on the glycemic index and the recipes are positively scrumptious. Browse through this group of cookbooks when you're at the bookstore.

As you continue to think "meat and vegetables" as you plan your meals, the concept will become second nature to you. And because you will be eating in alignment with the glycemic index weight-loss maintenance program for the rest of your life, meal planning and cooking will become easier and quicker.

Cooking Ahead

One of the glycemic index eating mishaps you want to avoid is arriving home very hungry and not having anything ready to eat. When you are very hungry, your body, mind, and entire being feels like it could devour a horse, but will settle for a loaf of bread or a box of crackers. You don't want this to happen.

Keep a good supply of low-glycemic snack foods in your home, and we don't mean just celery sticks. We mean fruit, whole-grain rice or pasta, a variety of

> **Thin-spiration**
>
> When you arrive home very hungry and feel like you could eat a horse, first pause and drink a large glass of water. This is relaxing and will help get your mind working properly so you can quickly find some suitable food to eat. If you need to wait a few minutes for the food to heat up, make a cup of herbal tea to sip while you wait.

vegetables, and meats and fish. A great way to do this is to cook ahead and have the foods ready to eat when you walk in the door. Such meals as zucchini lasagna, fresh cut veggies, al dente spaghetti with meat sauce, baked chicken breasts or drumsticks, barbequed pork ribs, or salmon salad can be waiting for you in the refrigerator.

Cookbooks

Go to the bookstore and purchase three or four comprehensive low-carb and low-glycemic cookbooks. By comprehensive, we mean cookbooks that include useful recipes for breakfast, lunches, dinners, and snacks. You'll find suggested menus in Appendix D and recipes in Appendix E.

Read through them and get a feeling for the ingredients and preparation methods. Make a note of which recipes you and your family will enjoy. Then cook and serve. Yes, you'll be experimenting, but that's the only way to learn new life-supportive skills.

If anyone else in the family likes to cook, ask them to prepare a special low-glycemic meal for the whole family. That way, others can also take ownership for preparing and eating these delicious meals.

Wrong Weigh

When selecting a low-glycemic or a low-carb cookbook, look for one that doesn't recommend the use of artificial sweeteners, especially aspartame. Or, if the rest of the cookbook seems terrific, simply ignore the recipes that call for artificial sweeteners.

Cooking for Your Family

Preparing meals for more than one person can be challenging even without glycemic index eating as a factor. So let's look at some of the ways to manage and negotiate meals for a partnership or a family:

◆ Before you start on your glycemic index weight-loss program, call a family meeting to discuss your new eating needs and theirs. Ask for support and also assure your family that you'll be keeping their food needs in mind as you eat according to the glycemic index.

◆ Most important is that the basics remain the basics. Meat and vegetables should work for everyone. If you have an avowed vegetarian in the family, he or she should have plenty of variety, but instead of eating high-glycemic processed foods, there are many choices of whole unprocessed foods, including some starchy vegetables and all the nonstarchy vegetables, whole unprocessed grains, and legumes. But meat and vegetables simply aren't negotiable for a person on a glycemic index weight-loss program. Other foods are. This doesn't mean that the other people in your life need to exclusively eat meat and vegetables. It just means that's what you will prepare for your own meals.

◆ Practically speaking, other family members need to be able to eat their favorite foods—even if those foods don't fit in your glycemic index weight-loss plan. If you have the fortitude and strength, you can cook the family's favorite high-carbohydrate and high-glycemic foods. For example, cook biscuits made with wheat flour at the same time you cook ham and eggs for everyone. You can let others eat toast for breakfast while you enjoy eggs and fruit. If you don't have the ability to avoid eating too much of the high-glycemic foods, you'll need to work out a different arrangement.

◆ There's nothing about low-glycemic foods that will hurt anyone's health, so you don't need to apologize for the foods you prepare and eat.

◆ If your family prefers, keep high-glycemic snacks on hand for them. Assign a special place in the pantry for the high-glycemic snacks, while you have your special place for low-glycemic treats.

◆ Prepare some whole-grain side dishes or "comfort food" recipes from low-carb and low-glycemic cookbooks to serve your family as well as yourself. You could find some real winners that please everyone.

◆ When the rest of your family wants to order takeout, such as pizza or Chinese food, be sure to order a large salad or vegetables for yourself. Then you can eat the meat from the food and pass on the pizza dough or sticky white rice. Basically, you can eat any takeout for a meal provided it contains animal protein such as meat or eggs and you can fix a salad, fruit, vegetable, or low-glycemic whole grain as an accompaniment.

Be patient and ask for patience from your family. Together you can work this out. There's always the real possibility that everyone's nutrition will improve because yours has.

Brown-Bagging It

You can pack any meal and take it to work, a meeting, or even your child's soccer game. Packing along food makes it easy for you to stay true to your low-carb weight-loss program. Here are some sample menus for any time of day:

◆ If you aren't hungry for breakfast before you leave for work in the morning, pack breakfast. You can pack protein foods, such as hard-boiled eggs, or meat and cheese rollups with low-glycemic foods such as plain yogurt, a small yam, cut vegetables, and fruit. If you have a microwave available at work, crack two eggs into a microwavable container and cover. When you're ready for breakfast, cook them in the microwave and eat. Add vegetables, a small amount of cold whole-grain, low-glycemic rice, or fruit as a side dish.

◆ For lunch or dinner, tote along any kind of main dish salad, such as a chef, Cobb, Caesar, or shrimp salad. Bring cold chicken or roast beef. Barbequed ribs work—provided you can wash your hands after eating. Add cut-up vegetables, low-glycemic whole-grain pasta, or fruit.

◆ For treats, pack some nuts, nut butters, olives, hard cheeses, moderate amounts (one third cup) of dried fruit, one or two pieces of fresh fruit, or larger amounts of cut-up vegetables. These are all reliably wholesome. The prepackaged tuna packs that contain tuna, mayonnaise, pickle relish, and crackers also work well for snacks. But hold the crackers and the candy mint— they're high-glycemic.

Wrong Weigh

Be sure that you don't eat yogurt as your breakfast protein. It doesn't contain an adequate amount of protein to meet your nutritional needs and stoke your fat-burning mechanism. A 6-ounce serving of yogurt contains about seven grams of protein. You need about 20 per meal.

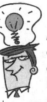

Thin-spiration

Meat and cheese roll-ups are simple and work for any meal or snack. Simply layer a piece of sliced meat with a slice of cheese and lettuce. Spread with mustard or one teaspoon of mayonnaise. Roll up and secure with a tooth-pick. You can vary the meats, cheeses, and condiments according to your tastes.

◆ Don't be caught without snacks for long car trips, outings, and excursions where you might not be able to find suitable food. Be prepared and eat well.

◆ Bring purified water with you to events so you can avoid sodas and sweetened beverages.

◆ Pack a packet or two of the electrolyte-balancing and energizing Emergen-C. Add to 8 ounces of water when you feel fatigued and need a quick and low-glycemic energy boost.

Taking along snacks and meals isn't just for people who are on low-glycemic weight-loss programs. Many people bring snacks and find them preferable to the high-sugar and high-glycemic snacks offered at ball games, festivals, and fairs.

The Least You Need to Know

♦ When planning and preparing meals based on the glycemic index, center them around meats and vegetables.

♦ Hold a family meeting when you begin your glycemic index weight-loss program to negotiate foods and family eating.

♦ Purchase some low-carb and low-glycemic cookbooks for meal and recipe ideas.

♦ Pack along low-glycemic meals and snacks when you're on the road.

Chapter 21

Special-Occasion Eating

In This Chapter

- Maneuvering special meals and emotions
- Eating at holiday meals
- Learning business-travel suggestions
- Vacationing the glycemic index way

When some people think of the holiday season, they immediately gain 5 to 10 pounds in their minds before Thanksgiving Day. Just thinking about the special holiday cookies, candy, and breads seems to predispose people to weight gain. And for good reason—for many, the holidays aren't as much about gift-giving as they are about eating.

What's a person to do who eats based on the glycemic index during the holidays? Refusing a second helping of pumpkin pie from Aunt Judy may be viewed as a personal insult. Simply announcing that you're watching your weight is an invitation for other well-meaning family members to urge you to eat more. Plus, your declaration of intended weight loss is likely to elicit comments declaring that you look anorexic and malnourished.

The holidays are challenging times for people who eat mostly low-glycemic foods, as are weddings, vacations, parties, and public events such as street festivals and ballgames. In this chapter, we guide you through the eating quandaries of all the special events in your life.

Your Inner Strength

Before we get into the details and specifics of eating at special events, you need to have an overall plan. Even people who have eaten unprocessed, lower-glycemic types of carbohydrates for years find it easy to slip up when eating at special events. It isn't so much that they lack willpower or self-control, it's just that the total environment is permissive and disorienting. They get into the flow of the moment, and the flow simply isn't in alignment with glycemic index weight loss. Before they know it, they've eaten a funnel cake topped with chocolate ice cream and syrup and washed it down with a high-fructose, corn syrup cola.

You've probably already experienced this, and you know how easy it is to get caught up into the frozen-chocolate-cheesecake-on-a stick mentality. Here's what it takes to enjoy an event without eating poorly in the junk-food or family-emotional flow:

◆ Stay conscious of your glycemic index weight-loss program. One of the joys of special events is that you enjoy being outside your usual life patterns. You get to have fun. But at the same time, you—as a person eating for glycemic index weight loss—need to remember your overall purpose in eating. That is, to eat more unprocessed, lower-glycemic carbohydrates, to continue losing weight, and then to maintain it.

◆ Ignore the fun junk foods. Cotton candy, Aunt Sara's fudge, blue sno-cones, Grandma's banana nut bread, and candy Easter eggs are part of your past, not your present.

◆ Always sit down to eat. No standing up or over the kitchen counter while eating.

◆ Don't overeat. Remember how awful you'll feel later if you overeat. You'll also feel awful if you eat that junk food now.

◆ Assume that no one else will understand your food needs and that you have to take care of yourself. Unfortunately, this includes close family members as well as street taco vendors.

◆ Focus on anything but food. Get in the flow of the event and ignore the food.

◆ Eat slowly and peacefully when you have the opportunity to eat low-glycemic foods. Think unprocessed, whole foods such as fish, poultry, meats, fruit, nuts and seeds, and vegetables at all eating opportunities.

◆ Keep a bottle or glass of purified water with you at all times. Make sure you don't get thirsty.

◆ Both willpower and self-discipline are highly reliable for short bursts of time. Gather these personality strengths before the event so they endure for several hours at a time. Use them to avoid high-carb foods and overeating, and to replace bad foods with your glycemic index weight-loss commitment.

◆ Don't let yourself get too tired, hungry, angry, or anxious. All these can trigger unnecessary eating.

Use all your internal resources to enjoy the special event. Learn to disassociate treat foods from specific events. In other words, hot dogs aren't a requirement for enjoying a ball game and pumpkin pie isn't going to make Thanksgiving any more complete.

Navigating the Holidays

You may be apprehensive about eating low-glycemic foods during the holidays and being faithful to your glycemic index weight-loss program. Your first low-glycemic holiday season is usually the most challenging. By the following year you'll know how to navigate the parties, family meals, and office treats with ease.

Holidays are times when you can enjoy these low-glycemic special foods:

◆ **Meats.** Roast turkey, smoked meats, baked ham, roasted pheasant, and game.

◆ **Fruit.** Some mail-order catalogs have beautiful fruit offerings.

◆ **Unshelled nuts.** These can be found along with fancy or plain nutcrackers in grocery and specialty stores.

◆ **Salted nuts.** Pecans, pistachios, and cashews, which can often be purchased from mail-order catalogs.

◆ **Unsweetened baked sweet potatoes and yams.** Eat in moderation, keeping in mind your daily carbohydrate allotment.

◆ **Imported specialty cheeses.** Both plain and smoked.

◆ **Vegetable trays.** Include nonstarchy vegetables such as celery, broccoli, cherry tomatoes, and cauliflower. Relish the good low-glycemic choices, but pass on the sweet pickles.

Be sure to take advantage of these wonderful low-glycemic holiday foods. Who says holiday foods are only about high-glycemic cuisine? Just be aware of the foods you need to avoid.

High-Carb Holiday Foods

The easiest way to deal with high-carb, high-glycemic holiday foods is to ignore them. They aren't going away, because many of those foods are part of our cultural heritage, but you don't need to eat them. Avoiding them isn't boring, it's wise.

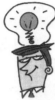

Thin-spiration

Ask yourself how you can best celebrate the holidays. What special gifts can you give to others? These can be actual presents, but can also include gifts of time and caring for others in special ways. This lets you keep food and eating separate from the season's true meaning.

Keep on thinking "meats and vegetables" when confronted with office goodies and family desserts, and learn to think differently about what the holidays mean.

It's easy for a person who loves food to focus on the eating aspects of the holidays, when, in fact, the holidays are far greater than the food. This year, focus on the people, the relationships, and your special religious observance. Think of the holidays as a time for good cheer and not just for good food.

Family Traditions

Eating with your extended family for holiday meals can be either wonderfully supportive or oddly confusing. If your family truly supports your glycemic index weight-loss efforts, appreciate the situation. Eating with them will be easy.

If your family doesn't understand your weight-loss desires, you're not alone. Sticking to your glycemic index weight-loss program is challenging when important family members have contrary opinions. Here are some suggestions for eating with extended family:

- ◆ Avoid discussing your glycemic index weight-loss program. If anyone notices you've lost weight, say "Thanks" and change the subject.

- ◆ Eat meats and vegetables. Eat additional foods only as your weight-loss phase permits. In other words, avoid eating high-carb, high-glycemic foods.

◆ If anyone asks why you aren't eating as much as they want you to eat, smile and tell them you: a) aren't so hungry; b) are really enjoying the meats and vegetables; c) are more interested in their new projects, vacations, and so on.

◆ Ignore any off-the-wall or unkind comments and then change the subject. Keep possible discussion topics in mind so you don't miss a beat.

◆ Remember that you are neither anorexic nor malnourished. You're simply thinner than they remember. Thank them for noticing.

◆ If family members are truly supportive and interested in your weight-loss success, have fun discussing your program and answering their questions.

◆ Ask others plenty of questions about themselves.

As best you can in this potentially disorienting environment, keep in mind the true purpose of sharing holiday meals with family. Enjoy their company, feel the love, and stay in good cheer.

Wrong Weigh

You should ignore your family's concerns about your weight loss only if you are carefully watching that your BMI (Body Mass Index) doesn't drop below 19. If it does, your weight could be too low and you need to stop losing weight immediately. Being too thin is unhealthy and dangerous.

Parties

Parties are so much fun, especially when you don't need to deal with the food. Usually the food is great, but you know you can't eat as much as is presented on buffet tables. In fact, you may be getting dressed for the party while wondering how you're going to eat mostly low-glycemic foods amid a sea of cookies, cakes, and bread-based appetizers. Here's how:

Wrong Weigh

Don't try to satisfy your carb-cravings with alcohol. If you choose to enjoy an alcoholic beverage, do so as you would normally do. Don't increase your alcohol intake during the holiday season.

◆ Don't start eating until you have reviewed all the food offerings. Zero in on the appealing low-glycemic foods and pass over any foods that don't look very appetizing.

- Talk to many people and put your energy into mingling and enjoying the people, not the food.

- Sip on club soda, mineral water with a twist, or empty a packet of Emergen-C into your soda. Add some ice and you have a vital, nonalcoholic, five-carbohydrate energy replenishment. For more info on Emergen-C, see Chapter 15.

- If you want a piece of wedding cake, have a taste. Ditto a toast of champagne.

- When appropriate, bring a hostess gift of delicious low-glycemic appetizers, such as deviled eggs or sliced ham with fresh vegetables and condiments. Also add some acidic condiments such as dill pickles or marinated vegetables.

On Vacation

Some people actually lose weight on vacations. They relax so much that their cortisol levels drop. They can then release built up stored fat. Lucky them.

Other people gain weight on vacations. This is the situation for most people. But by eating wisely, you can continue your weight-loss progress while on vacation. Here's how:

- Don't eat continental breakfasts—even when they're free—unless they offer meats, cheeses, fresh fruit, or eggs. Otherwise, you'll be eating free high-carb and high-glycemic foods. Instead, go to a restaurant for breakfast, or if you can, prepare breakfast yourself.

- Keep your alcoholic beverage consumption the same as at home. Don't drink more than usual.

- Get enough sleep. Don't try to stay up too late every night, because your body could start to store more fat.

- Keep on thinking and eating meats and vegetables.

Body of Knowledge

If you vacation at a vegetarian-style resort, you'll find it difficult to eat adequate amounts of complete proteins without also eating foods high in carbohydrates. If you absolutely must vacation at such a resort, bring along packages of tuna, sardines, and some hard-boiled eggs so you can eat the foods you need to support your weight loss and your health. While at the resort, eat fresh vegetables and fruit and pass on the high-glycemic foods.

◆ Don't go long periods of time without food or water. Plan to eat every four to six hours, or even more frequently depending on your body's specific needs.

◆ If you're in a foreign country with native cuisine quite unfamiliar to you, such as India or Thailand, bring along some familiar foods that you already enjoy, such as peanut butter, dried fruit, tuna, and shelled nuts.

> **Thin-spiration**
>
> Cruises offer plentiful food virtually all day and all night long. Be selective in your food choices and don't get caught up in simply eating because the food is available. It's time to practice being discerning and picky. Take advantage of the plentiful exercise and excursion opportunities on board and off.

By following the previous guidelines, you'll be able to at least maintain your weight on the trip and quite possibly continue your weight loss.

Business Travel

Eating while traveling on business is challenging when on a low glycemic weight-loss program. Any time your body rhythms are disrupted, you are more likely to gain weight and less likely to lose weight. Jet lag is a foe of dieters everywhere. But some simple guidelines can help you maintain steady weight loss with a business-travel lifestyle.

◆ Keep up your exercise program and stick to it faithfully. Fortunately, most hotels have exercise rooms and many offer fully equipped health clubs. Be sure you're up and at 'em early enough to take advantage of the fitness center. Pack your gym shoes and exercise clothes first.

◆ Airline food is now nonexistent, unless you're traveling first class or very long distances. If you want to eat when flying coach, bring along your own food. You can purchase good main-dish salads from the airport concessions and also fresh fruit. If you have time, eat a sit-down meal at one of the airport restaurants, keeping in mind to order foods such as meats, chicken, fish, vegetables, and fruit.

◆ Pack foods and snacks for times when you won't be able to sit down and eat a meal. Bring along cans or packages of tuna, dried fruit, shelled nuts, natural beef jerky, a baggie of fresh-cut veggies, and cheese. Some hotel restaurants will provide sack meals for breakfast, lunch, and dinner.

◆ At business dinners, continue to eat as recommended on your glycemic index weight-loss program. If you're famished, start with a low-glycemic appetizer and not with the bread basket.

◆ Because adequate sleep helps with weight loss, do your best to have a good night's sleep. If necessary, pack some creature comforts. Some people pack their favorite pillow, scented bath oil, music, or reading material to encourage a good night's sleep.

All the previous tips will help forestall an energy crash when your body's natural rhythms are out of sync—a fattening energy crash. If you have other favorite travel comforts, be sure to incorporate those into your business-travel plans.

At the Festival

Some special events offer up plenty of fun and plenty of fast food, but virtually no low-glycemic foods. We're talking about ball games, art festivals, jazz festivals, carnivals, state fairs, circuses, and many other enticing outdoor summer attractions.

You may be strolling along and all of a sudden the luscious aromas of waffle cones or the sight of freshly baked pretzels is too much to resist. What's a mostly low-glycemic eater to do? In addition to the enticing aromas, you'll see lots of people snacking and eating as they enjoy the full experience. You'll want to do the same thing.

Well, to put it bluntly, you can't take it all in. At least not the foods. You need some strategies:

◆ Find a food vendor that offers foods that are low-glycemic and/or low-carb. For example, a pulled-pork sandwich—hold the bun—with a side of vegetables is actually a good low-glycemic offering. Even a hot dog works fine if you can forego the white-bread bun. A chicken taco salad, hold the tortilla, is also good low-glycemic fare. In addition to protein food and salads, corn-on-the-cob on a stick or fresh fruit might also be found at outdoor food vendors. Both of these are also low-glycemic.

◆ Stay away from the booths that offer the high-carb/high-glycemic snacks. Curiosity can easily kill a weight-loss plan.

> **Body of Knowledge**
>
> Theaters offer the following treats as you sit ringside watching a hilarious comedy: pizza, french fries, popcorn, pretzels, and breadsticks. What would you be ordering? Water. Eat before you go to the theater and enjoy the show *sans* the high-carb foods.

◆ Keep bottled water close at hand.

◆ When you're hungry and want to eat a meal, find a restaurant, if possible, and sit down to eat.

◆ Don't get too hot and sweaty without electrolyte replenishment. Your body wants water and minerals, but your instincts could be to eat as a means of replenishment. Carry electrolytes with you when you anticipate sweating in the hot sun. See Chapter 15 for recommendations on electrolytes.

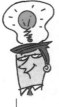

Thin-spiration

Here's how to eat hot dogs or brats without the bun. You can use a fork and knife, but if that's too messy when eating on your lap, order the hot dog with the bun. Then, holding the bun in one hand, eat the end of the meat, and then slide the meat forward and eat the meat that's sticking out of the bun. Continue until all you're holding is the bun and the meat's all gone.

Taking actions to prevent hunger and thirst frees up your energy to enjoy the fair or festival while you continue to lose weight down to your ideal size and then maintain it.

The Least You Need to Know

◆ You can find ways to eat low-glycemic foods at virtually any party or special event by eating meats, fresh fruits, and vegetables.

◆ Carry low-glycemic snacks on vacations and business travel for the times when low-glycemic foods aren't readily available.

◆ Gather your inner strength for sharing special meals with family and naysayers.

◆ At special events, focus your energy on the people and the purpose of the party and not on the food.

Quick and Easy Snacks and Treats

In This Chapter

◆ Finding quick low-glycemic snacks

◆ Eating at sporting events

◆ Finding convenience-store snacks

◆ Overcoming continental breakfast challenges

What do you do when you're hungry for something and you're not sure what it is? In the past, you may have scrounged through the pantry and refrigerator searching for that something that would satisfy your craving. Mostly likely it was a high-glycemic snack—just what you didn't need.

While it's relatively easy to order a meal for glycemic index weight loss or to prepare one at home, it's generally more challenging to figure out what to eat for snacks.

In this chapter, we give you plenty of suggestions for low-glycemic snacks for home and other places. You'll find foods you can prepare and eat in and also some that you can carry with you when you are away from home.

What's in a Snack

Your ideal snack is easy to make or quick to find. But you need to be prepared for when a snack-attack hits. So fill your pantry and refrigerator with these low-glycemic treats for yourself and your family:

◆ **Stuffed dates.** Fill dates with ¹/₂ teaspoon of plain cream cheese or with an almond or pecan. Eating 3 to 4 gives you a glycemic load of 10. Any date lover will think "yummy!" Not familiar with dates? Start treating yourself!

◆ **Meat and cheese rollups.** Roll up a thin slice of meat and a slice of cheese in a lettuce leaf. Secure with a toothpick. Have 1 or 2. There's no glycemic load. None! But, there are calories in the form of fat grams, so be sure to keep meat and cheese amounts within the limit for the day.

Body of Knowledge

Daily protein recommendations for women are no more than 9 ounces of lean meat, poultry, fish, or an equivalent protein, and no more than 1 ounce of cheese per day. For men, it's no more than 12 ounces of lean meat, poultry, or fish and no more than 1 ounce of cheese per day. Equivalent protein foods include foods such as cottage cheese, eggs, and egg whites. Three fourths cup of cottage cheese equals the same amount of protein as 3 ounces of meat. If you eat whole eggs, then substitute 2 whole eggs for 3 ounces of meat.

◆ **Plain whole fruit with a cup of herbal tea.**

◆ **Snow cones.** Although it's best to eat whole fruit rather than fruit juice, for a treat, make a snow-cone. Purchase a snow-cone maker at a kitchen store—they cost about $19.95. Fill the container that comes with the snow-cone maker about one third full with unsweetened juice or ¹/₄ cup juice, top with water, and freeze. When you want a snow-cone, the snow-cone maker will churn out an icy treat in less than a minute. The glycemic load is about 3.

◆ **Pickled eggs.** You can find these at food specialty stores and at the deli. Make your own with the recipe for pickled eggs in *The Complete Idiot's Guide to Low-Carb Meals*. Even just one makes a filling snack. The glycemic load is 0.

◆ **Hard-boiled eggs.** They're an easy snack. Just keep a few in the refrigerator. The glycemic load is 0.

♦ **Cut up vegetables with dip.** For snacks, cut some vegetables into snack-size pieces when you arrive home from the grocery store. That way, they're ready for munching when the urge hits. When eating them raw isn't appealing, you can dip them in vinegar and oil salad dressing, a full-fatted dressing, or a lower-fat dressing. The glycemic load for all these is close to 0 per serving.

♦ **Nuts.** You can choose from any kind of nuts you enjoy—macadamias, pecans, almonds, hazelnuts, peanuts, and pistachios. A serving size is 6 to 10 nuts. You can eat them salted or spiced. You can find recipes for spiced nuts in many cookbooks. Just be sure that the topping doesn't contain sugar. They have no glycemic load.

♦ **Cashews.** Although these nuts are low-glycemic, they do contain a few more carbohydrates and thus have a slightly higher-glycemic load. Three tablespoons of cashews have a glycemic load of 3.

> **Thin-spiration**
>
> You can combine several of these suggestions into one snack. For example, you can eat a hard-boiled egg, a dried apricot, and 1 stone-ground low-glycemic cracker. Or enjoy a 1-ounce cube of cheese with a quarter slice of low-glycemic stone-ground bread.

> **Wrong Weigh**
>
> Be sure to measure out the amount of nuts you eat. It is easy to munch unconsciously and overeat. Eat slowly and you'll find that any snack becomes more satisfying and enjoyable.

♦ **Parmesan crackers.** Picture a wafer of pure toasted Parmesan cheese. They're yummy and make a great party snack. You can make these ahead and enjoy them when you need a snack. Preheat your oven to 375 degrees. On a cookie sheet, spread one 6-ounce package of shredded Parmesan cheese into a thin layer. Bake for about 10 to 12 minutes or until melted and slightly browned. Cool slightly, then remove the toasted Parmesan from the cookie sheet and just break it into pieces. One or two pieces make a great anytime snack. The glycemic load is 0. A serving is 1 ounce.

♦ **Low-glycemic crackers and breads, such as pumpernickel rye kernel bread.** One ounce has a glycemic load of 5. Have 1 or 2 crackers or 1 ounce of bread. Suggestions for toppings include flavored mustard, a small slice of cheese, or 1 teaspoon of nut butter.

◆ **Homemade trail mix of nuts, seeds, and dried fruits such as dried apricots and cranberries.** A serving size is 3 tablespoons. The glycemic load ranges from 1 to 2.

◆ **Olives.** There are many varieties of delicious black olives or green olives. Eat 3 or 4 for a snack. The glycemic load is 0.

◆ **Cocktail onions.** Two or three make a nice snack. The glycemic load is 0.

◆ **Half of a small avocado.** Remove the pit and eat with a spoon. You can also fill the "hole" of the avocado half with salad dressing, such as vinegar and oil, Italian, or Ranch. Put the pit in the other half and wrap. Place in the refrigerator and eat within a couple days.

◆ **Guacamole salad.** Prepare with ½ avocado, cut into cubes. Toss with lime juice, salt, and a sprinkle of chili powder.

◆ **Sliced fruit such as apples, oranges, and pears.** One half of one of these fruits has a glycemic load of 2 to 3.

◆ **Nut butters on fruit slices.** Use ½ tablespoon of peanut or almond butter on about 2 ounces of fresh fruit slices such as pears or apples. The glycemic load is about 2 to 3.

◆ **A mustard-tasting party.** Purchase several different flavored mustards and serve on cut-up vegetables such as jicama, celery, and carrots. Vegetables with enticing mustard makes a tangy snack that satisfies your need for crunchy and sour-tasting foods. The glycemic index is 0, with no fat.

◆ **Beef or meat jerky.** Purchase jerky that doesn't contain mystery ingredients. You can find it at a natural-foods store or some specialty stores. (The convenience store varieties have enough chemicals in them to seem like you're back in chemistry class! Yuck.) Or make your own. The glycemic index is 0. As a bonus, jerky is low in fat.

◆ **Small cans of tuna or sardines.** Eat the tuna plain or mix with a small amount of mayonnaise. Purchase sardines in mustard or tomato sauce and eat right out of the can with a fork. When eaten plain, there's no glycemic load.

◆ **Dark chocolate.** Even a small square of chocolate makes a great snack. Rather than chew it, let the square dissolve slowly in your mouth. You'll derive great pleasure for a very low-glycemic load of about 2. One 17-gram dark chocolate bar is considered 1 fat serving.

◆ **Unsweetened fresh coconut.** A chunk or two makes for a fun snack for coconut lovers. There's no glycemic load, but coconut is a fat.

◆ **Raw carrot sticks with fresh ginger and a cup of ginger tea.** The glycemic load is 3 for 1 cup of carrots or 1 medium carrot.

◆ **Small baked yam ($\frac{1}{2}$ cup).** Top with plain yogurt (2 tablespoons). The glycemic load is 6.

◆ **Steamed fresh green beans (2 cups) lightly sprinkled with Parmesan cheese.** No glycemic load.

◆ **Hot blended green drink.** Cooked fresh beet or spinach greens with the cooked vegetable water, $\frac{1}{2}$ ounce of feta cheese, and $\frac{1}{4}$ cup of cottage cheese. Blend after cooking for a warm revitalizing drink. This drink is very filling and tastes great with no glycemic load!

◆ **Low-glycemic food bars.** Some food companies such as USANA have several low-glycemic food bars. Their ingredients are natural with no artificial sweeteners.

In addition to these snacks, go through the lists of low-glycemic foods in Appendix B and look for combinations that are appetizing and appealing to you. Always be sure that your snacks are within your daily glycemic load allotment.

Snacks on the Run

If you've ever tried to find low-glycemic snacks at a convenience store, undoubtedly you either walked out in frustration or you gave in and ate a high-glycemic treat. Seems that convenience stores are little more than high-glycemic food filling stations. And the same holds true for the office snack machine and the snack counter at the movies. In this section, we give you some palatable suggestions for finding snacks at the most unlikely places.

◆ **Convenience stores.** If you're lucky, the convenience store has a bin full of fresh fruit, including apples or pears. If so, go ahead and purchase this sweet treat. If they don't have something fresh, you can probably find a snack of trail mix

Wrong Weigh

At the convenience store, you won't find low-glycemic treats on the candy shelves, inside the donut box, or nestled alongside the pretzels and chips. So don't even bother looking there. Why let yourself be tempted to blow your plans for a healthy, lean body?

made with nuts, seeds, and dried fruit. Or you might find some suitable beef jerky. However, most brands of beef and meat jerky are filled with chemical preservatives and mystery ingredients, so read the labels as carefully as you can and choose the jerky with the fewest mystery ingredients. You may also be able to find string cheese or unsweetened yogurt.

◆ **At the movies.** The snacks at movies are generally high-glycemic. We can't recommend the candy or popcorn. Most likely the best you can do is bottled water. Eat before you leave home. Better yet, bring a low-glycemic treat in your purse or coat pocket. (It really is okay.)

◆ **Lunch wagons.** Hopefully you'll find some fresh fruit and sandwiches and maybe pickled eggs or cheese. If the sandwiches are made with white or whole wheat bread, you may need to hold the bread and eat the insides of the sandwich. Or only eat $1/2$ piece of bread. Pickles and mustard are fine. Use lunch wagons as a last resort; instead, pack your lunch to take to work.

◆ **Office vending machines.** If the vending machines are stocked with only high-glycemic foods, you can petition the supplier for better food choices. Ask for small packets of nuts, trail mix, and fruit. Otherwise, steer clear of this part of the lunchroom and bring your own late afternoon snack from home. Items such as dried fruit can be kept in your desk drawer for a long period without going bad.

◆ **The coffee shop.** Perhaps you're meeting a friend for morning coffee or a late afternoon latte or cappuccino and you'd like a snack as well. Unfortunately, the snacks at coffee shops are usually baked goods made with white flour. They look scrumptious but are hardly low-glycemic. Some coffee shops offer exquisite dark chocolate bars. You could purchase one and eat 1 or 2 squares.

◆ **At the ballpark.** Peanuts and crackerjacks are the trademarks of baseball games. Yes, enjoy the peanuts, but hold the crackerjacks. If you attend major or minor league sporting events, you already know what the food is like. To say the least, it doesn't fit in well with your glycemic index weight-loss program. This doesn't mean you need to give up the games but that you need to become very clever about the eating. Today, most ballparks don't let you bring in your own food. So you're stuck with the food concession offerings. Choose hot dogs, brats, or hamburgers, but forego the bun. Purchase salads when you can find them. Pass on the sugary soft drinks, and instead, buy bottled water or juice. Even though juice has generally a relatively high-glycemic load, it does have some nutrition and you can limit the amount. You can tuck a pre-packed mozzarella cheese stick in a pocket or purse to eat with diluted juice. A small glass of beer could be acceptable if you're so inclined.

♦ **Continental breakfasts.** You find these at conventions and other types of meetings. Usually they offer Danish pastries, high-glycemic breakfast cereals, bagels, butter, cream cheese, milk, juice, fruit, coffee, and tea. Slim pickings for your glycemic index weight-loss program. What's missing is an adequate amount of animal protein. If you are stuck eating at a continental breakfast, choose fruit and several packets of unsweetened cream cheese. This should hold you for an hour or two.

> **Thin-spiration**
>
> If you are planning an event or business meeting with a continental breakfast, consider asking the chef to offer hard-boiled eggs or some cold cuts of meats along with the standard fare. You'll find the meeting participants have more sustained energy and enthusiasm to carry them through to lunch.

We predict that you'll find low-glycemic food offerings more widely available as soon as the popularity of eating based on the glycemic index grows. Until that time, be prepared. Carry along low-glycemic snacks to events, on airplanes, and to meetings. Keep some snacks in your glove compartment and your desk at the office.

The Least You Need to Know

♦ Keep low-glycemic snacks in your pantry and refrigerator for when you need a quick snack.

♦ Carry low-glycemic snacks with you so that you'll always have something on hand to eat.

♦ Eat discriminately at sporting events and the movies.

♦ Don't rely on convenience stores, coffee shops, and lunch wagons for low-glycemic food offerings.

Part 5

Insulin, Cortisol, and Weight Loss

Insulin and the stress hormone cortisol are intimately connected, and both affect your weight-loss success. The less stress you have, the lower your insulin levels. The reverse is also generally true. The lower your insulin levels, the lower your stress. When you learn how to reduce your stress on a daily basis and keep it low, you'll find that losing weight, and especially losing weight through your midsection, is easier and, better yet, the weight stays off.

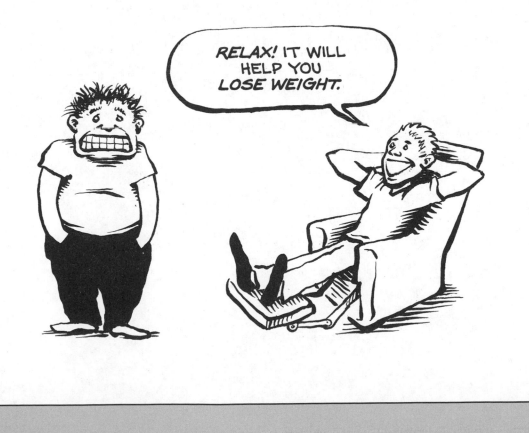

23

Breaking the Insulin/ Stress Cycle

In This Chapter

♦ Understanding the stress cycle

♦ Knowing cortisol's role in weight gain

♦ Avoiding cortisol-inducing foods

♦ Lowering your stress load

Let's say you have one of those weeks when your stress levels skyrocket. You face a major life-changing event. Your workload increases substantially although the hours in your week remain the same. Your energy levels were already low and dealing with normal, day-to-day stress puts you over your comfortable stress limit.

Then, at the end of the week, you step on the scales and find you have gained weight. Unfair! So unfair! After all, you were absolutely faithful to your glycemic index weight-loss eating program.

Glyco Lingo

Cortisol is a stress hormone secreted by the adrenal glands that stimulates the release of glycogen stores in the liver and in the muscles. Glycogen is the body's storage form of carbohydrate that breaks down into blood glucose in times of need. The extra blood glucose produced by cortisol increases stamina, endurance, and mental acuity during times of stress.

How can it be? What went wrong?

First of all, you didn't do anything wrong. Your glycemic index weight-loss program didn't fail you. Blame the stress. Stress all by itself can cause weight gain even if you're faithfully eating according to the glycemic index.

The reason is that your body's stress hormone, *cortisol*, plays a significant role in insulin function, which in turn impacts your weight. In this chapter, you learn how stress affects your insulin levels and how insulin affects your stress levels. The hormones cortisol and insulin play off each other and can make you a gainer or a loser, based on how cleverly you eat and manage your stress.

Your Body's Stress Cycle

Stress just *is*. It is part of our lives, and it just isn't going away. Your body's response to stress is hard-wired directly into your biology to protect you. For instance, your body gives you a burst of energy when your safety is threatened. Your body's response to stress is actually very important to your well-being—that is, unless you live with chronic day-to-day stress and have no means of escape.

When stress becomes unrelenting, it becomes seriously detrimental to your well-being. Too much ongoing stress can lead to heart disease, diabetes, depression, mood disorders, high blood pressure, cancer, and other diseases and health disorders. Notice that these are the same chronic health conditions that can be caused by hyperinsulinism and insulin resistance (more on the similarities in a moment).

For now let's explore how your stress cycle works. The first phase is the excitation phase. This is triggered by an event that turns on your flight-or-fight response. The trigger event can be as simple as a loud and unexpected noise or the sudden news of a tight deadline at work. Your body likely secretes the stress hormone adrenaline. It can happen in a flash. Your heart pounds a bit faster, your reflexes become more sensitive, and subconsciously you become physically on alert to fight or to flee.

During the second phase, immediately after your body secretes adrenaline, your adrenal glands secrete the stress hormone cortisol. Think of cortisol as control central. Cortisol gives you stamina, energy, and courage, as well as the mental edge to make quick decisions and to resolve the situation. Cortisol remains in your bloodstream until the stressful event comes to an end.

Body of Knowledge
Even our ancient ancestors experienced serious stress, but in general, they could decompress more easily because their stress triggers weren't as unrelenting as ours are today. Imagine a caveman being chased by a wooly mammoth. His adrenaline starts pumping. He knows he has to take action or risk death. Cortisol kicks in and gives him the energy and stamina to make a quick getaway and duck into a cave to hide. Scary, yes! But when the caveman is out of danger, his body begins to recover as he relaxes. The cortisol level in his body decreases. Although you and I might not want to live the lifestyle of a caveman, at least he got to relax! Many of us find ourselves in high-stress cortisol-inducing situations day in and day out. It's hard on the body.

After you have dealt with the stress, your body enters the third phase: the recovery phase. Your pulse rate returns to normal, the stress hormones are metabolized out of your body, and life calms down. In an ideal world, you cruise along easily until you encounter another big stress trigger.

In today's world, the three-phase stress response seldom has a clear beginning, middle, and end. Often a person doesn't complete one stressful event before another one starts. As a result, many people experience ongoing stress that never seems to stop. They have many irons in the fire at one time, and their cortisol levels never drop completely. Instead, their cortisol levels stay elevated day after day and year after year, leading to weight gain and insulin resistance and eventually to chronic health disorders.

The Insulin/Stress Connection

The link between insulin and cortisol is complementary. When insulin levels rise, so do cortisol levels. When cortisol levels rise, so does insulin. In other words, chronic elevated insulin levels can increase your stress levels. Stress increases cortisol, and the more cortisol in your body, the higher your insulin levels.

Insulin is sometimes referred to as a *storage hormone*. It's responsible for keeping your blood sugar levels within a narrow range. It also functions to store fat in your cells, to store sugar in your liver, and to influence amino acids used for muscle building.

But when you're under stress, you need your energy released from storage so that you can use it. Cortisol commands your body to do this by directing it to, essentially, ignore insulin's direction and instead to make sugar, fat, and amino acids available for conversion into glucose. When the amino acids are pulled from your muscles for energy, your muscle mass decreases.

Thin-spiration

Public awareness and some of the scientific information about the intimate link between the levels of insulin and cortisol is relatively new. So stay tuned. As researchers dig further, they'll find more ways to help you manage your weight and your stress levels as the link between these two powerful hormones is better understood.

Cortisol commands your cells to stop uptaking sugar, which increases the insulin in your bloodstream. At that time, cortisol is directing your cells to be insulin-resistant.

Likewise, when your insulin levels are too high, as when a person's blood sugar levels are low, the body will secrete cortisol in an attempt to release glycogen stores in the liver to increase the blood glucose levels. When a person is insulin-resistant, and has too much insulin in the bloodstream, the body secretes more cortisol to balance the effects of too much insulin.

In essence, your body's stress hormone, cortisol, causes weight gain.

Cortisol-Inducing Foods

Overuse of some foods and medications causes your body's cortisol levels to increase. And guess what? Many of the foods are the same that directly increase your blood sugar levels, and ultimately, your body's insulin levels. Those foods are the following:

- Caffeinated beverages, such as coffee, sodas, black tea, and green tea
- High-glycemic starches and sugars
- Beer, wine, and other alcoholic beverages
- Too many grams of carbohydrates or too high a glycemic load eaten at one time
- Caffeinated foods, such as chocolate
- Herbal stimulants, such as bitter orange and ephedra, which was recently banned for consumption by the FDA
- Foods that you are allergic to or that you have a sensitivity to

Right now, you aren't eating high-glycemic starches and you're limiting your total carbohydrate intake, so you're already avoiding some foods that raise cortisol levels.

But if you find that your weight loss seems to be stalled or that you're gaining weight, then cut out caffeinated beverages and foods along with alcoholic beverages.

It seems that everyone has a different tolerance level for these cortisol-inducing foods. If you notice that a cup of coffee makes you jittery, hold the coffee and instead drink a beverage that's more soothing, such as an herbal tea or even hot water.

On the other hand, if a taste of chocolate within your carbohydrate levels is more soothing than enervating, go ahead and luxuriate in its taste. For some people, a little is fine, but too much puts them into cortisol overload, and most likely, carb overload, as well.

> **CAUTION**
>
> **Wrong Weigh**
>
> They don't call them beer bellies for no reason. Alcoholic beverages stimulate cortisol production, which leads to fat storage in the midsection—in the belly. This occurs whether the alcoholic beverage does or does not contain carbohydrates.

Weight-Loss Stress

Here's the rub: Even the mere fact that you're on a glycemic index weight-loss program is stressful. You're trying to be more vigilant about everything you eat. You're making lifestyle changes, which produce more stress, even though they're positive changes. Even the foods you eat are different.

You're also monitoring your changes in weight, which is also stressful.

Yuck! Does this sound like you're caught in a vicious cycle? You're right. The cycle goes like this: The more stress, the more cortisol running through your body. The more cortisol, the harder it is to lose weight and the higher the possibility of insulin resistance. Insulin resistance causes weight gain.

But wait! There is a solution to this.

Other people have been highly successful losing weight on a glycemic index eating program, which means you can, too. The easiest way out of the vicious cycle is to accept that during your glycemic index weight-loss program, you'll have more stress initially, but that will subside after you eliminate stress triggers in other areas of your life. You also need to find time daily to reduce your cortisol levels through stress-soothing activities. We discuss those techniques in Chapter 24. After it becomes a habit to eat the glycemic way, your stress level will decrease.

Eliminating Stress Triggers

It's time to make a quick "stress analysis" of your life to figure out which stress triggers you can eliminate.

Certainly, many of your stressors can't be eliminated, but if you can let go of even a few, you may see immediate results as weight loss become easier. Here are some suggestions:

◆ Avoid rush-hour traffic on your way to and from work. Leave earlier or later to avoid high-stress traffic. For the long term, if you drive long distances to work every day, you may want to consider moving to a new location or finding a job that's closer to your home.

◆ If you're already stretched thin at work with an excessive workload, just say "no" when asked to take on more responsibility for outside activities, such as volunteer organizations or civic groups.

◆ If watching the news is distressing, turn it off.

◆ For the duration of your glycemic index weight-loss program, try to avoid making major life decisions such as marriage, divorce, job changes, increasing the size of your family, home remodeling, or other life-changing situations.

◆ Try meditation. Persons who consistently meditate at least once a day can find it easier to lose weight.

After you've eliminated as many stress triggers as possible, the stress triggers that remain are the ones you need to live with. But you can do something about them, too. That information is in the next chapter.

The Least You Need to Know

◆ When you're stressed, the stress hormone cortisol causes an increase in your body's insulin levels.

◆ Elevated levels of cortisol over time can lead to insulin resistance and weight gain.

◆ Chronic hyperinsulinism can increase your stress levels by increasing your body's cortisol levels.

◆ Eating based on the glycemic index combined with stress reduction can increase weight loss and ease weight-loss maintenance.

24

Glycemic Index Weight-Loss Aids

In This Chapter

- Preventing high cortisol levels
- Using daily stress soothers
- Finding a "crafty" way to de-stress
- Using cortisol-reducing supplements

Picture yourself coming home from work or another activity in the late afternoon or early evening. The day has been long and tiring, and your nerves are frayed. You search through the kitchen cabinets looking for a low-glycemic food—heck, any food!—that will mend your nerves. Nothing seems right.

But before you can relax, all the demands of the evening begin. You need to toss in a couple loads of wash, cook dinner, and then monitor the children's homework. You can't fathom finding time just for yourself. Even the notion of eating your dinner in a beautiful environment seems a remote luxury.

This situation is *not* conducive to weight loss, but what can you do? You don't need a pep talk about eating broccoli instead of cookies. You need a stress soother that reduces your cortisol levels, at least for the rest of the evening.

Don't despair! In this chapter, you discover many ways to reduce your cortisol levels and, simultaneously, reduce insulin levels so that you can more easily lose weight and maintain your weight loss. You'll be able to stop the vicious and fattening cortisol-insulin cycle.

Daily Cortisol-Management Program

The best way to manage your stress level is to control your body's stress response before it controls you. By using an ounce of prevention, you can keep your cortisol levels lower all day long. You just need to follow a three-part program that's easy to manage. And it will be especially easy for you because you're already doing two of the three parts.

This cortisol-management program is great because it works for everyone. Trust us, it will work for you:

♦ Eat the low-glycemic way. Don't skip meals. When you eat carbohydrates, make sure they're low-glycemic. Avoid starches unless they're low-glycemic. By doing this, you're avoiding cortisol-inducing foods. Also, don't consume foods or beverages containing caffeine or alcohol. Avoid products containing bitter orange or other nervous system stimulants.

Glyco Lingo

EPA, eicosapentaenoic acid and **DHA,** docosahexaenoic acid, are considered to be the most important omega-3 essential fatty acids. They are only found in animal products, especially deep-water fish such as salmon. They help rev up your fat-burning mechanism.

♦ Take fish oil or flaxseed oil every day. The essential fatty acids in the oils help with brain function by regulating chemicals called prostaglandins. If these prostaglandins are disrupted, it can cause anxiety, depression, and mood swings. Research shows that fish and flaxseed oils can reduce symptoms of stress and soothe feelings of aggression and hostility. Plus they aid in brain neurotransmitter functions. Research studies have been done on fish oil and flaxseed oil. In order for flaxseed oil to be as effective as fish oil, a person's body needs to be able to convert ALA (alpha lineoleic acid) into adequate amounts of *EPA* and *DHA*. EPA and DHA are present in fish oil, but not in flaxseed oil. If your body can't convert the flaxseed oil or you suspect that it can't, you should take the fish oil. If you want to be sure that you receive adequate amounts of EPA and DHA, you should choose the fish oil.

Most adults can take about 1 teaspoon to 1 tablespoon of fish oil or 4–12 capsules of fish or flaxseed oil per day. Be sure you don't purchase fish liver oil, but instead pure fish oil.

◆ Do vigorous aerobic exercise at least three times a week for 45 minutes. It will help get your heart rate up high enough for you to literally sweat. Taking a walk around the block is not going to work unless you walk or jog fast enough to sweat. If you prefer, you can do vigorous sweaty aerobic exercise for 20 minutes every day. Vigorous exercise increases the flow of endorphins in your body and makes you feel good.

Wrong Weigh

If you suffer from gallbladder or digestive problems related to fat metabolism, you may need to use only 1 teaspoon of oil or only a couple of the capsules initially and then see if you can gradually work up to more.

Wrong Weigh

If you ever gain weight or reach a plateau in your glycemic index weight-loss program, make sure that you're following your program correctly, including aerobic and strength-training exercises. Then reduce your cortisol levels with some of the stress soothers explained in this chapter.

By following these three steps, you'll better handle the stress that comes your way. You'll be able to handle stressful situations without experiencing as much internal stress yourself.

Thin-spiration

Emily called herself high-strung. Unlike the motto "don't sweat the small stuff," she did. She felt as if navigating life was like walking through a minefield. Her body size varied with her stress levels. Then she began eating the low-glycemic way and using the daily cortisol-management program. She was no longer on pins and needles after work. She could more easily handle the day-to-day chaos of raising a family and sustaining her marriage. Everyone involved breathed a big sigh of relief when she stopped sweating the small stuff.

Of course, some days are harder than others. When confronted with new or more intense stress triggers, you'll still experience a rise in cortisol levels. That's why you need additional stress soothers to help you manage all the stressful events in your life.

Stress Soothers

Some good news to remember: You can lower your cortisol levels without dramatically changing your life. You can keep your job, your family, and all you hold dear. But you will need to start incorporating stress reducers into your lifestyle.

Today researchers know what reduces stress because they can measure it. Researchers can now measure a person's cortisol levels with a saliva test. You might be a bit surprised by some of the results.

In one study, researchers tested the cortisol levels of a group of individuals. Then the test subjects hung out on the sofa to rest and relax. After an hour, the researchers retested the subjects and their cortisol levels hadn't changed. Seems sofa time is *not* a particularly good de-stressor. They then had the same group do one hour of yoga. The cortisol retest showed a significant reduction in cortisol levels. Whoa. Yoga actually fulfilled its promise of soothing ragged nerves. What's interesting is that the very thing that a person would think of as relaxing—just lounging on the sofa—wasn't effective.

So, here's a list of activities that are effective for reducing cortisol levels.

Get in Water

Warm water soothes your skin, which is the largest organ in your body. A warm-to-hot bath before dinner or before bed may be all you need to lower your cortisol levels and feel renewed. As you lie in the tub, imagine all your stress flowing from your body into the water and then down the drain. After your water break, put on some fresh clothes and enjoy the rest of the evening. If you bathe right before bed, then snuggle into the covers and let yourself drift off to sleep.

You can get soothed in water in the hot tub, bathtub, shower, or even a swimming pool. Your immersion can be very short. Even 5 to 10 minutes may be all you need to relax.

You can make your bath more soothing and sensuous by adding bath salts, fragrant essential oils, or Epsom salts. Two all-time inexpensive favorites are sea salt and baking soda.

Get Some Sunshine

Experts tell us that we need at least 15 minutes of sunshine or bright light every day for our hormones to function optimally. Remember that cortisol and insulin are hormones, as are our reproductive hormones.

The best way to receive this blessing from the sun is to spend at least 15 minutes outdoors. Here are some simple options:

◆ Eat your lunch outside

◆ Work in your garden

◆ Take a walk

Be sure to use sunscreen, but it's actually better if you avoid wearing sunglasses with UVA and UVB protection because your eyes need to be exposed to the light for that 15 minutes. (Just a safety note here: Don't look at the sun; instead, simply be in the sunlight.)

You may want to use a light box if the day is cloudy or overcast, or if you live in the northern part of the country where the sun doesn't shine much in the winter. These boxes are about the size of a laptop computer and they put out very bright light. Many people use them to remedy SAD, seasonal affective disorder. You can find one online by doing a keyword search for "light box."

Sunshine perks up your mood and helps you manage stress more easily.

Stretch Your Body

As you proceed through the day and your stress increases, your muscles tighten and contract. When you stretch, the muscles release the tension. This is one of the reasons yoga is so effective at reducing cortisol levels.

So learn how to stretch and then stretch any time you need a refreshing break. You can stretch at the office, after your shower in the morning, after work, or right before dinner. Generally, it's easiest to stretch on an empty stomach.

You can learn the correct ways to stretch by taking yoga classes or stretching classes. Or read one of the many stretching or yoga books available. A classic stretching book is by Bob Anderson, called *Stretching*. Plus you can find videos on stretching at www.collagevideos.com. An Internet search will turn up lots of possibilities.

The rules for stretching are quite simple:

♦ **Be gentle.** Don't force your body into a posture; instead, let your muscles open up to the stretch.

♦ **Go slow.** Take your time. Stretching works better if you're moving slowly.

♦ **Be patient.** Over a period of several months, you'll be amazed at your new flexibility.

Thin-spiration

Yoga enthusiasts believe that as a person's body gains more strength, balance, and flexibility, those same qualities are incorporated into the person's life and way of being. Who couldn't use more internal balance, strength, and flexibility?

Stretching is also incredibly affordable. You really don't need any special equipment at all. Wear clothing that lets you stretch—either loose clothing or stretchy pants and tops designed for yoga. Consider purchasing a sticky mat that offers padding and prevents you from slipping. Beyond that, all you need to do is just do it!

Personal Pamperings

Ahhh, those massages, facials, manicures, and pedicures. All of them can significantly reduce your cortisol levels. If you can afford them, by all means, pamper yourself and reduce your stress level at the same time. Some individuals find that a massage helps them stay stress-free for a week or two.

If you can't afford these spa-type treats, then use the following personal pamperings that cost merely pennies per use or are totally free:

♦ Find ways to trade pamperings with a friend or spouse. For example, trade foot massages. Even 10 minutes of a foot massage goes a long way to relax you.

♦ Use a back roller. Check out the Maxi-Backsie at www.bodytools.com. It costs about $25 and lasts forever. And it's highly relaxing. A back roller looks like a wooden rolling pin but with waves in it. To start, place it just below your neck. As you relax, your body weight will help the tool work deep into the erector muscles along the spine. Then slowly move the tool down your back, breathing about 5 to 10 times at each vertebra. By the time you reach the lowest part of your back—after about 15 minutes—you'll be wonderfully relaxed. The back roller relaxes the erector muscles on either side of your spine and massages acupressure points and lymph glands along the way. Use the back roller anytime you need to de-stress. There is also a handy one to use for traveling or when sitting down.

◆ Use a still-point inducer. You can find one online at www.gaiam.com. It costs about $25 and lasts forever. Just lie down with your upper neck-lower scalp on the inducer. Lie still for 5 to 10 minutes and let the inducer's gentle pressure create the "still point," a quiet pause in the rhythm of the craniosacral system. Users claim that when the still point is reached, many beneficial and therapeutic effects as well as deep relaxation occur. Some people prefer to listen to soothing music while using the still-point inducer, but it works wonderfully when used in silence.

◆ Try body rolling. Find information about this highly relaxing method of body alignment at www.yamunabodyrolling.com. Body rolling uses balls ranging in size from a couple inches to about 8 inches in diameter. Spend a half hour rolling down your thighs, up your back, or on your feet and you'll feel great. Body rolling is also used for body realignment, because it works somewhat like deep-tissue massage. We think it helps eliminate cellulite. The cost for the beginner kit is $49.

With a little imagination, you'll discover many other forms of personal pampering. When you find one that works, use it often to keep your cortisol levels low and your mood calm and even.

Brush Your Hair

It almost seems too simple to be true: Brushing your hair is both relaxing and good for you. Many women have intuitively known this for years. Brushing your hair helps get your stress hormones back in balance. The best hairbrush to use is a very inexpensive one that has plain plastic bristles that are rough on the tips, which stimulate your scalp better. The hairbrushes with rounded plastic tips may not work as well.

To brush your hair, bend over from the waist and brush, making sure that the bristles are reaching through your hair to your scalp. Brush for a minute or two, then stand up and rearrange your hair. You'll feel great—refreshed and energized.

You can brush your hair anywhere that you have a brush and a private area. Yes, restrooms work just fine for this.

Arts, Crafts, and Hobbies

Hobbies are healthy. Well, at least many of them are. An activity that shifts you out of work mode, or life-maintenance mode, into a world of creativity, rhythm, or beauty will help you tackle everyday stress. The hobby that you enjoyed as a young person may be the same one that brings you relaxation and a sense of serenity today. Of course, the list of possibilities is endless, but here are some ideas for getting started:

- Handicrafts, such as knitting, crochet, needlepoint, sewing, or quilting
- Visual arts, such as sketching, painting, photography, sculpture, scrapbooking, or pottery
- Gardening
- Woodworking, home repair, rebuilding cars
- Playing a musical instrument
- Writing letters, poems, novels, articles, and journaling
- Puzzles, such as crossword puzzles and jigsaw puzzles
- Leisurely reading
- Games, such as bridge, scrabble, and monopoly
- For some people, cleaning, ironing, or house-painting are stress soothers

It seems amazing that so many highly enjoyable activities reduce your cortisol levels. But don't get out of control with your hobby. Yes, you can be productive and also reduce your stress levels, but don't let your fun activity create more stress. In other words, do your arts, crafts, and hobbies as leisure activities and not with deadlines and urgency. Otherwise you're likely to create more stress.

Meditation and Prayer

Many persons have had huge success with reducing cortisol levels through a process known as "stilling the mind." Research studies show that individuals who meditate regularly, meaning once or twice a day, experience better sleep, lowered blood pressure, and decreased risk of cardiovascular disease and stroke.

If you are interested in pursuing meditation or prayer as a means to reduce stress, you have many choices. For centuries, people have used prayer, contemplative prayer, and meditation. The basic technique for meditation is to sit still for 20 minutes twice a day, preferably morning and late afternoon. The meditator focuses on a mantra, which is a series of simple syllables, and repeats the mantra aloud or silently while breathing in and out. That's all there is to it. It sounds simple, but it can create profound calm. Contemplative prayer is similar.

You can learn to meditate on your own by using a meditation tape or by simply reading a book on meditation and doing the suggested exercises. Or you can take a meditation class. Many classes are offered through extension centers at universities and community colleges. You can also take courses on prayer and contemplative prayer through your church or place of worship.

> **CAUTION** **Wrong Weigh**
>
> Researchers have yet to determine whether playing video games reduces cortisol levels. We know that watching television isn't a reliable stress reducer. Until you hear otherwise, don't expect video games to reduce your cortisol levels.

Other Stress Soothers

Use these additional stress soothers to maintain a lifestyle and attitude that lowers your stress level:

- **Positive thinking.** You can use motivational tales and books as well as spend time with inspiring people. Many people find religion and religious activities valuable for many reasons, and one is to reduce stress.

- **Spend time with friends.** Build healthy relationships. Believe it or not, a healthy bonded relationship by itself can reduce stress.

- **Listen to pleasant music.** Even houseplants are healthier when listening to beautiful sounds. You will be, too.

- **Use aromatherapy.** Yes, it's true. Breathing in the scents of essential oils can calm you down. You can also use a couple of drops in bathwater for a stress-soothing bath. Try lavender, clary sage, spruce, jasmine, or rose. Or choose another fragrance that smells great to you.

- **Get adequate sleep.** Most people need about eight hours. Don't settle for less sleep than you need. Otherwise, your stress levels could soar.

You may have other stress soothers that work well for you. When you find one that works, use it when needed. Not only will you feel great and happy, you'll also be supporting your weight-loss program.

Stress-Soothing Supplements

Recently some nutritional supplements have been shown to reduce cortisol, and they've been finding their way to health-food store shelves. So check them out and, if they work for you, use them either daily or when you're feeling highly stressed.

Some of these supplements are advertised as helping with weight loss. They can be a partial answer to avoiding insulin resistance and the ensuing weight gain, but they aren't the total answer for attaining one's ideal size.

◆ Green tea contains compounds, especially theanine, which are calming. If you can handle the caffeine in the tea, you can drink as many as 3 cups a day. If the tea hypes you up, you need another choice.

Thin-spiration

Before you stock up on cortisol-reducing supplements, be sure you're taking the basic nutritional supplements recommended in Chapter 16. Many of them, such as the B vitamins, calcium, and magnesium, provide you with the extra nutrients you need when stressed.

Wrong Weigh

Use caution when taking these cortisol-lowering nutritional supplements. Some may work well for you and others won't. Record when you use these in your food diary and also write down any positive or negative results. That way, you can find the combinations that work best for you.

◆ Theanine alone can help control stress. It's an amino acid found in green tea leaves, but you can purchase it in capsules at any health-food store. Theanine relaxes you without sedating you. In fact, theanine helps increase your brain's production of alpha waves, the brain waves associated with alert thinking and reasoning. No known adverse side effects have been reported. You can use theanine daily or when needed, but don't take more than 200 mg per day. You'll feel its effects within a half hour and the relaxation lasts for about two hours. We don't recommend that you take theanine before bed, because it increases your mental alertness and to sleep you need to turn off your active brain.

◆ Epimedium is an herb that comes from an ornamental bush grown in Asia and the Mediterranean. In research studies, epimedium extract reduced blood levels of cortisol and improved immune system function. Be sure to purchase water-extracted epimedium, because it has shown no adverse side effects. You can use up to 1000 mg per day for cortisol control.

- Phytosterols are found in fruits, vegetables, nuts, and seeds, which means you're consuming them now, right? They modulate your immune function, reduce inflammation and pain, and help control allergies. They also reduce cortisol levels. You can also purchase phytosterols as a supplement, but we encourage you to get all or most of these phytosterols from food. If you do want to take a supplement, taking between 100 and 300 mg per day of a mixed phytosterol blend that includes beta-sitosterol is the recommended amount.

- Magnolia bark helps control cortisol levels and is beneficial for lowering anxiety and stress. However, if you take too much, you could experience drowsiness or sedation. Some minor side effects have been reported, but it's generally considered safe. Purchase magnolia bark to prepare as a tea or in pill form. You can take between 250 and 750 mg per day.

- 5-HTP (5-hydroxytryptophan) is a form of one of the essential amino acids, tryptophan. Tryptophan converts in the brain into serotonin, which can help improve mood, decrease appetite, and improve sleep. Initially start with a small dose (30 to 50 mg) on an empty stomach, preferably in the late afternoon or before dinner. Don't take 5-HTP with food because it's not effective then.

> **CAUTION — Wrong Weigh**
>
> Don't use 5-HTP every day, but rather use it once every other day or about three times a week. Taking the supplement too often can cause some of the same side effects as the SSRI antidepressant medications. These include Prozac and Zoloft.

> **Body of Knowledge**
>
> Read the label carefully. Some of the supplements can be taken regularly, up to three times a day. Others may work best when used on an as-needed basis.

Don't use all the previous supplements at the same time—that's way too much. Start with one and determine if it works for you. If not, try another one. Stop if you have any negative reactions. Hopefully, you'll find one or two that work well for you.

You can find stress formulations at health-food stores that combine several of the previous supplements into one pill. You'll need to experiment to find a formula or product that works best for you (see Appendix C).

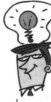

> **Thin-spiration**
>
> When using these stress-soothing supplements, you may want to take some three times a day, about eight hours apart. This can help your moods stay balanced because you'll have some in your body throughout the day. A reminder can be to take them at meals.

The science of cortisol-control through supplementation is new, and you can expect more news and more supplement formulations as research progresses. As more people use these for cortisol control, expect more reported side effects and more information on how they work in the body. Before you use any of these supplements, do further research on the Internet to read about possible side effects and usage recommendations.

Weight-Loss Supplements

You've read the ads and watched the infomercials about the latest weight-loss supplements. Perhaps you've tried them but down deep in your heart wondered if they were first of all, effective, and second of all, safe to use.

Products that contain ephedra, a thermogenic enhancer, have been pulled from the shelves by the FDA. A similar ingredient, bitter orange, is on the FDA watch list, but as of now is still used in many products.

Now there's a new fat-loss product and delivery method that could be helpful. The fat-loss patch delivers reliable and consistent amounts of Forslean, chromium, and guarana. Forslean comes from the coleus forskolii plant, which is grown in Asia. It's effective and safe for gentle weight loss. It works through an entirely different biological mechanism than both ephedra and bitter orange, which both stimulate the adrenal glands. Forslean supports the thyroid gland, which regulates your metabolic rate. Chromium helps regulate blood sugar levels and preserves lean muscle. Guarana contains caffeine just like coffee and tea, but delivers only 1.2 mg of caffeine per hour, which is quite low compared with a cup of strong coffee, which contains between 100 and 120 mg.

Consider using the fat-loss patch if you are eating based on the glycemic index and doing regular and frequent exercise. It may aid you in moving beyond a weight-loss plateau and in controlling your cravings for high-glycemic foods. You can learn more about the patch at www.nexagenusa.com/bethinpatch.

The Least You Need to Know

- Use the daily cortisol-management program to keep cortisol and insulin levels low.

- Take time daily to decompress and relax using one of the stress soothers.

- Develop an interest in arts, crafts, or hobbies that will help you manage stress and lower your cortisol levels.

- Cortisol-reducing supplements work to chemically reduce your cortisol levels and assist with weight loss.

Chapter 25

Toxins and Glycemic Index Weight Loss

In This Chapter

- ◆ Releasing toxins
- ◆ Learning the functions of the liver
- ◆ Using glycemic index weight loss to reduce toxins
- ◆ Managing your body burden

Most people cringe when they learn their bodies are filled with toxins. Just the thought that more than 100 toxic chemicals are present in the average person's body seems … well … it seems unbelievable. But that's not all. Those toxins can block your body's ability to release stored fat.

A person with a higher toxin load can have a more difficult time losing weight. Fortunately, a glycemic index weight-loss program helps the body flush toxins and promotes eating healthful foods that don't contain more toxins. And it's good for people with average toxin loads as well.

Glyco Lingo

Toxins are chemical substances that harm or irritate the body. A person can get toxins into the body through breathing, consuming them when eating, drinking, or taking medications, and through skin contact.

Wrong Weigh

Some health experts believe that too many toxins in the body can lead to more fat storage. They surmise that the body will actually conserve fat and possibly create even more fat in which to store the toxins rather than let the person be poisoned.

In this chapter, you learn how toxins play a role in weight loss and how low-glycemic eating helps you release the toxins that normally tend to prevent weight loss.

Your Toxin Load

We all have *toxins* in our body. There's nothing anyone can do to avoid getting at least some toxins inside the body. We acquire toxins from the foods we eat and the air we breathe. Toxins are absorbed through the skin from skin lotions, sunscreens, and household cleaners.

Toxins can be either water-soluble or fat-soluble. Water-soluble toxins are stored in water-based body fluids, such as lymph fluid and blood. Fat-soluble toxins are stored in body fat.

By storing the toxins away from major body organs, your body is protecting you from being poisoned. Actually, this is rather ingenuous, when you think about it. But losing body fat reduces your body's toxin-storage capacity. This presents a challenge for weight loss.

Toxins Stored in Fat

As your body uses stored fat for energy, the toxins that were stored in the fat are released into your bloodstream, tissues, and organs. Because toxins are poisons, this sudden flooding can make you feel awful. You can feel irritable or experience headaches, nausea, and lightheadedness.

Do you recall how you felt during the first couple weeks of a previous weight-loss program? Most likely, you didn't feel all that great. If you're like most dieters, you attributed that run-down feeling to being deprived of the foods you loved. Certainly that could have been the reason for feelings of emotional deprivation. But in truth, toxins were flooding your system and making you feel under the weather.

Major sources of toxins include the following:

◆ Environmental pollution that you breathe, including car exhaust and gasoline fumes

◆ Second-hand smoke

◆ Medications, including over-the-counter medications

◆ Poor-quality drinking water

◆ Pesticides and herbicides

◆ Paint, carpet, and household cleaner fumes

◆ Some skin creams and topical ointments, such as bug spray and sunscreens

You can't avoid all the previous sources, but you can minimize your exposure to them as much as possible. When you do, you lighten what's known as your *body burden*, the amount of toxins that your body has to deal with.

The Liver as a Detoxifier

Your liver is the organ that manages two important functions as you lose weight. First, your liver converts stored fat into energy. This is what makes glycemic index weight loss so effective. Your body uses stored fat for energy rather than glucose from carbs. You want your liver to be in tip-top form to perform this important function.

The second function of the liver is to process out body toxins. All toxins go through the liver on their way out of the body. Toxins can

Thin-spiration

We applaud cities that have banned smoking in all public buildings, including restaurants, bars, and nightclubs. Plenty of toxins already exist in the air we breathe, and no one needs to add to his or her personal toxin load by breathing in someone else's cigarette or cigar smoke.

Glyco Lingo

Body burden denotes the amount of toxins that an individual has within their body at any point in time.

Wrong Weigh

A high body burden of toxins has been indicated as the cause of serious disease conditions such as cancers and autoimmune diseases. As you ease your body burden and help promote toxin flushing from your body, you may experience other important health benefits.

be eliminated through sweat, urine, feces, breath, and mucous. But they don't get there until they first go through the liver.

The liver works based on priorities. First it processes out toxins, and then it converts fat to energy. If its workload of toxins is too high, it may not get to its lower-priority jobs, such as converting fat into energy. Yes, that means you won't lose weight as fast.

It's to your benefit to keep your body burden low so that you can lose weight faster and more efficiently. You can do this by avoiding the following foods and beverages:

- ◆ **Alcohol.** You've heard that drinking too much alcohol over a lifetime can destroy liver function through a disease called cirrhosis of the liver. What you may not know is that even a drink or two takes energy away from your weight-loss efforts because the liver needs to detoxify all alcohol a person drinks.

- ◆ **Chemical food additives.** These are the kinds you are avoiding on your glycemic index eating program. These include food colorings, preservatives, and artificial sweeteners. Avoid foods that contain these "mystery" ingredients.

- ◆ **Caffeinated drinks.** Too much caffeine from such foods and beverages as coffee, black or green tea, kola nut, guarana, chocolate, cocoa, colas, and some over-the-counter pain medications, in addition to affecting cortisol levels, prevents proper hydration, thus making it harder for the body to eliminate the toxins.

- ◆ **Sugars.** To adequately metabolize calories, the body needs nutrient-dense foods. Empty calories cause an excess burden on the body.

- ◆ **Trans-fats.** You are already avoiding foods that contain partially hydrogenated oils because they are harmful to your health. Because they are harmful to your body, they require detoxification by your liver.

- ◆ **Diets low in fiber.** When you eat for glycemic index weight loss, you are eating plenty of fiber. Don't ever return to a low-fiber diet.

- ◆ **Foods high in saturated fats.** Some foods high in saturated fats can contain more toxins such as PCBs (polycholorinated biphenyls). Therefore, be sure to cut excess fat from meats and poultry, and be selective when purchasing fish.

As you can see, by eating low-glycemic foods you are actually helping your liver convert stored fat into energy because you're lowering your body burden.

> **Body of Knowledge**
>
> To avoid the PCBs in fish, buy fish that is harvested away from the inland and farther out into the ocean. Farm-fed salmon is an example of a higher-fat, inland-harvested fish, so avoid eating it. To prevent consuming mercury found in ocean-going fish, avoid swordfish, shark, and king mackerel, and limit canned tuna to one serving twice a week. Keep your saturated fat intake to no more than one third of your total fat intake and you'll reduce your risk of ingesting toxins found in saturated fat. On the glycemic index weight-loss program, you eat about one third of your fat from polyunsaturated fats, one third from monounsaturated fats, and one third from saturated fats.

Removing Toxins

The previous recommendations help you avoid adding to your body burden by avoiding the sources of toxins. But you can go even further and actually help reduce your body burden by helping your liver function well and by helping the process of flushing toxins from your body. To do this, follow these tips:

- Eat plenty of vegetables and fruits. Veggies and fruits contain antioxidants, which neutralize the free-radical damage that can be caused by toxins. They also include plenty of fiber, which helps move toxins from the body through the bowels. Aim for 25 to 50 grams of fiber a day.

- Avoid highly processed foods and junk foods. Generally speaking, these contain a lot of toxins. Read the ingredient list and you'll find food colorings, chemical preservatives, and plenty of ingredients that are impossible to pronounce. If you assume the unpronounceable ingredients are toxins, you'll probably be right about 90 percent of the time.

- Eat essential fatty acids in your foods and take an essential fatty acid supplement. The good fats help remove toxins from the body.

- Drink at least eight glasses of purified water every day, perhaps more. Water flushes out water-soluble toxins and also the fat-soluble toxins that have been converted by the liver to water-soluble ones.

- Exercise. Exercise is wonderful for supporting all metabolic functions, including the liver's function. Exercise lets you sweat out the toxins.

♦ Take antioxidant nutritional supplements to go along with your antioxidant-rich vegetables and fruits. Toxic substances trigger inflammatory prostagladins. Antioxidants help protect against the free radicals that occur due to this inflammatory process.

To avoid the run-down feeling when toxins are being flushed from your stored fat, be sure to follow the previous recommendations during your entire glycemic index weight-loss program.

Obviously, avoiding toxins is a good lifelong goal for general health. Toxins add unnecessary and unwanted stress on your body. Because you'll be eating based on the glycemic index indefinitely *and* avoiding toxins, you'll get a double benefit: a great-looking body and a healthier one.

The Least You Need to Know

♦ Toxins are stored in body fat and are released when a person loses stored fat through weight loss.

♦ During weight loss, the released toxins can cause headaches, irritability, and fatigue.

♦ As best you can, avoid increasing your body burden or toxin load by making lifestyle changes.

♦ By following a glycemic index weight-loss program *and* avoiding toxins, you can lose weight and boost your overall health.

Part 6

The Exercise Advantage

Exercise for weight loss isn't just about burning calories. The effects of exercise on your body's biology can enhance your weight-loss efforts. Use aerobic conditioning, strength training, and stretching or flexibility training to propel your body to release stored fat. Of course, you'll also enjoy the great shaping, toning, and postural benefits of your daily exercise regimen.

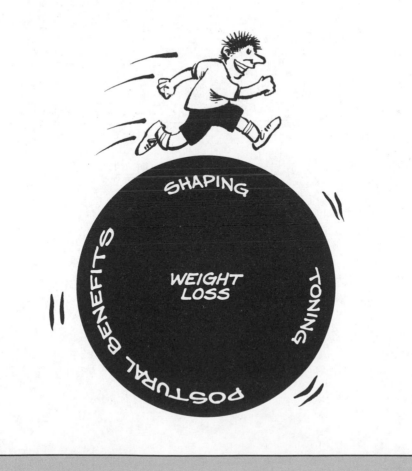

SHAPING

POSTURAL BENEFITS

WEIGHT LOSS

TONING

Chapter **26**

Give Your Body Movement

In This Chapter

- ◆ Using aerobic exercise
- ◆ Reducing insulin resistance
- ◆ Creating an aerobic conditioning program
- ◆ Getting started

Now it's time for the fun part of glycemic index weight loss to begin. You've already read about the biological and medical reasons for eating based on the glycemic index. You know what to eat and what not to eat. We would love to tell you it's going to be lots of fun, but you know it's going to require lots of attention and, quite honestly, some sacrifice. Thank goodness the results are worth it.

This is why exercise is going to seem so easy to you. You already know how to move your body. You know it makes you feel great. You know that the very fact that you follow an exercise program is a status symbol, making you the envy of your couch-potato friends. As an added bonus, exercise can be fun. Compared to the effort initially required to change your eating habits, it's easy to master exercise.

Of course, you need to actually do it. That is, you need to lace up your athletic shoes and get a move on. In this chapter, we tell you what types of exercise your body craves and how to satisfy this amazing hunger.

Aerobic Exercise

The first type of exercise your body hungers for is aerobic exercise. This form of exercise is now often referred to as cardio, which is short for *cardiovascular*. Whatever you choose to call it, you should do *aerobic exercise* to increase your heart rate for at least twenty minutes three times a week. By the end of the twenty minutes, you should be sweating. Okay, women are supposed to glow and the guys sweat. Call it whatever you choose, but be sure to do it.

> **Glyco Lingo**
>
> **Aerobic exercise** can be any type of exercise that you do for a sustained amount of time, at least fifteen minutes, that moves your major muscles and makes you huff and puff and break into a sweat. Running, jogging, swimming, and bicycling are popular forms. But vigorous hiking, racquetball, tennis, or dancing are also considered aerobic exercise, as are aerobic conditioning classes. Golf, bowling, and billiards aren't.

You have many choices for aerobic exercise, such as jogging, biking, running, and swimming.

> **Body of Knowledge**
>
> Perhaps you've read or heard that doing such activities as heavy housework and gardening is an adequate substitute for aerobic exercise. Quite simply, it isn't. Yes, those types of activities are great for you and your body, but they're seldom able to give your heart the endurance it needs. So do your housework or gardening, but be sure to add a regular aerobic exercise routine. In this situation, the more aerobic exercise you do, the better.

Aerobics and Insulin Resistance

Aerobic exercise is an important factor in supporting your weight-loss program. The biological benefits serve to enhance the health benefits of the glycemic index.

Vigorous aerobic exercise increases your cells' ability to absorb glucose. This is important if you have insulin resistance, hyperinsulinism, or diabetes. Here's why: When a person is insulin-resistant, the body's cells refuse to obey the insulin's commands to absorb glucose. This means that too much insulin stays in the bloodstream and that blood glucose levels are elevated.

Elevated levels of insulin and glucose mean that your body stores the glucose as fat and you gain weight. Insulin resistance can also lead to diabetes.

When you do cardio exercise, you actually improve the entire insulin-glucose-carbohydrate cycle, making it more efficient. Although this mechanism isn't exactly about losing weight, the ultimate result of reducing or eliminating insulin resistance is a change in the way your body uses energy and stores fat.

When your insulin levels are lowered, so is your level of the stress hormone cortisol, so aerobic conditioning can help reduce stress—both long-term and short-term.

Just reading this information must be making you want to lace up your shoes and start moving. But before you do, there are still more weight-loss benefits to cardio exercise, so read on.

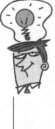

Thin-spiration

If you feel sluggish, fatigued, or are bombarded with carb cravings, aerobic exercise may be the answer. Even a couple minutes can perk up your metabolism and energy levels and energize your cells, because they'll be getting an extra boost of glucose. If you eat carbohydrates when you're sluggish, fatigued, or plagued with cravings, you could experience weight gain and lowered energy levels while increasing the cravings.

Aerobics and Fat

Aerobic exercise burns fat. You already know why. It takes energy—namely calories—to fuel your body. During aerobic exercise you need plenty of fuel to burn. When you're eating for glycemic index weight loss, your body burns stored fat for fuel.

The primary sources of fuel for aerobics during a glycemic index weight-loss program are carbohydrates and fat. When you first start exercising, your body uses glycogen stores (your body's form of carbohydrate) for fuel. After those are used up, the body uses fat. Now that you're eating fewer carbohydrates, you have less glycogen stored, so your body begins burning stored fat sooner in your workout. What an unexpected bonus!

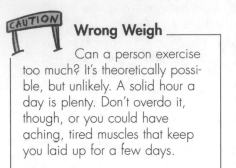

Wrong Weigh

Can a person exercise too much? It's theoretically possible, but unlikely. A solid hour a day is plenty. Don't overdo it, though, or you could have aching, tired muscles that keep you laid up for a few days.

If you weren't eating based on the glycemic index, your body wouldn't use as much fat as its fuel source. An added bonus of continuing your exercise program is this: The more trained a muscle is, the greater its ability to use fat as fuel. Exercising regularly and consistently increases your fat-burning capacity. The result is that it's easier to stay at your ideal size.

Also, the length of time of your exercise sessions pays off. Any amount of aerobic exercise burns fat, but of course, the longer you exercise, the more fat you burn.

Aerobics and Your Heart

When a person has insulin resistance, the excess insulin causes the body to store fat. The initial form of fat stored is called triglycerides. Yes, these are the same triglycerides that contribute to high levels of LDL. This type of cholesterol is the kind that clogs arteries.

When you do aerobic exercise, you reduce insulin resistance, thus reducing your body's inclination to increase triglyceride storage. At the same time, you increase your body's good cholesterol, called the HDL level. The HDL, or high-density lipoprotein, helps carry away excess cholesterol.

That's the first piece of good news. But there's more. Aerobic exercise strengthens your heart muscle and its pumping efficiency. Aerobic exercise is a gift to your heart. And, because your heart is the core of your body, it's a gift you give to yourself.

Aerobics and Your Moods

You've heard about the runner's high, which happens when a person's endorphins are released and make him or her feel absolutely great, uplifted, and sometimes enlightened. You also know that low levels of serotonin and other brain chemicals can lead to feelings of depression, anxiety, and carbohydrate cravings.

What you may not know is that you can use aerobic exercise to boost your moods. Exercise increases the good-feeling brain chemicals that annihilate those carbohydrate cravings while making you feel good. Yes, this is all totally legal, widely available, and better yet—free.

Aerobics and You

By now you are excited about the upside of aerobic exercise and are facing the same challenges that everyone ever devoted to a sedentary lifestyle faces. You can only reap the rewards if you physically start to move.

First of all, you have to, absolutely have to, ignore your own objections, complaints, justifications, and excuses. And you need to adopt the best exercise slogan ever written—Nike's "Just do it."

Then you need to decide what you're going to do. Here are some of your choices:

> ### Body of Knowledge
>
> Before you embark on a new exercise program, especially if you are out-of-shape and unaccustomed to exercise, check with your doctor. Also, if you start experiencing excessive pain or fatigue, seek professional health care and advice.

- **Stationary bike.** We love this because we can read while we pedal away for twenty minutes in the morning. Plus, if you purchase a stationary bike, you can exercise at home. You can also watch television while pedaling. Stationary bikes are great if you have weak or damaged knees that limit your ability to jog or use the treadmill.

- **Jogging or running.** If you can jog or run, go for it. Wear sunscreen. Start slowly and then increase distance and speed. Your basic equipment is nothing more than a good pair of running shoes and socks.

- **Swimming.** Make sure you like getting wet and then find a pool, lake, or ocean. Other than a body of water, all you need is a swimsuit. Swimming is great if you're just beginning to exercise or if you have lots of aches and pains that could preclude other kinds of impact exercise.

- **Cardio machines.** These include elliptical trainers, treadmills, and stair-steppers. Most fitness centers offer these along with a television to help you while away your aerobic minutes.

- **Walking.** Only choose walking if you're just beginning to do aerobic exercise. You'll benefit initially because you'll be moving. But after several months, you'll need to pick up the pace to continue receiving benefits. The best way to walk is to make sure that your heart rate is at the correct level for your age. (We discuss this later in this chapter.) Strolling isn't the same as walking. Think quick, brisk, fast, huff and puff.

Wrong Weigh

Avoid the stair-stepper if you were born with larger thighs. Instead of making them thinner, you could actually increase both their strength and size. Instead, choose another type of aerobic exercise. Intense stretching exercises could help make them smaller. We talk more about stretching in Chapter 28.

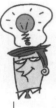

Thin-spiration

An added benefit of outdoor aerobics is that you can revel at being out in nature, enjoying the fresh air, and spending some time in the sun. Just be sure to wear sunscreen and bring along bottled water.

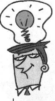

Thin-spiration

You can mix and match your aerobics. Perhaps you hike for two to three hours on the weekend, attend an aerobics class on Monday after work, and pedal on your stationary bike at home in the mornings before work. No matter how you combine your activities, do at least twenty minutes three times a week. More is better.

♦ **Aerobic classes.** Offered at fitness centers, these classes are designed to keep your heart rate up for at least forty-five minutes to an hour. Not only will you be moving to the music, you'll be gaining strength from calisthenics and other exercises. Be sure to attend class two or three times a week. You'll find many variations of aerobic classes, ranging from African dance to cardio yoga.

♦ **At-home videos.** You'll find a wide variety of aerobics videos online at www.collagevideo.com. These are a great choice if you like to exercise at home and really will slide the tape into the DVD player, push Play, and do the exercises. They're excellent for bad-weather days and very convenient.

♦ **Recreational aerobics.** Do you enjoy playing court sports such as racquetball, squash, or tennis? If you can play for an hour at full speed ahead, then these games can be excellent for aerobic conditioning. But if you like to talk through the game and take it easy, find another way to get your heart rate up.

♦ **Outdoor aerobics.** If you love the great outdoors, you can do your aerobic conditioning outside. Hiking, mountain biking, snowshoeing, and cross-country skiing are all excellent for aerobic conditioning.

♦ **Contact sports.** If you love basketball, volleyball, football, soccer, and other contact sports, go for it. These sports require skill, agility, and a certain toughness. Be sure you develop the required toughness before you play intensely. You absolutely don't want to be sidelined with injuries. You want aerobic conditioning to be fun.

◆ **Other gym equipment.** Yes, you can use other types of gym equipment for your cardio exercise. Just be sure to elevate your heart rate for a minimum of twenty minutes three times a week. More is better, but it's best not to overdo it.

Your Heart Rate

Now that you're doing aerobics, you're technically an athlete. As such, you need to be concerned about the quality of your conditioning. It only makes sense that you want to exercise in the best way possible.

In aerobic conditioning, your heart rate counts. Here are guidelines for the minimum, moderate, and maximum rates for your age.

Age	Minimum	Moderate	Maximum
20	125	145	165
30	120	138	155
40	115	130	145
50	110	125	140
60	105	118	130
70	95	110	125
80	90	103	115

While you're exercising, take your pulse to determine your heart rate. Some machines give you a real-time readout of your pulse rate. If you don't have an electronic readout, here's how to take your pulse:

1. Find your pulse. You can find it on the inside of your wrist or at the side of your neck just below and in front of your ear.

2. Wear a watch with a second hand. Count your pulses for six seconds and multiply by ten. That's your heart rate. If you want to be more precise, you could count your pulses for ten seconds and multiply by six. In either case, you get close, and that's all you need. If this doesn't appeal to you, you can purchase a heart monitor from a sporting goods company and use that.

In the midst of your session, your heart rate needs to be near the moderate number or above it. That means you're working hard enough. It's fine if your heart rate is higher than that, but don't exceed the maximum for your age unless you are in great shape. But if you are, you probably already know how to monitor your heart rate.

This is what you need to know: If your heart rate isn't high enough, your aerobic training isn't doing you much good. Yes, working out properly means you'll huff and puff and that you'll sweat. So be prepared.

If, however, you can't catch your breath, slow down. Check your heart rate and make sure it isn't too high based on the preceding chart. For the best results, keep your heart rate at a level where you can still converse while exercising.

Aerobic Do's and Don'ts

Use these helpful hints as you embark on your aerobic training. Success and pleasure breed more success and pleasure. Because you'll be participating in aerobic conditioning for the rest of your life, here are some ways to boost your success quotient:

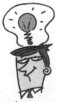

Wrong Weigh _____

You don't need to ease up on your aerobic exercise program as you start your glycemic index weight-loss program. Continue to suit-up and show up. Don't decide to sit at home instead of exercising. This will lead to bad habits, and you don't want that.

Thin-spiration _____

If your feet are blister-prone, wear two pairs of thin socks when you exercise. Also, if you can predict the location of blisters, put a Band-Aid on the spot before you put on your socks and shoes. Always break in your athletic shoes before a big event or pack along a second pair just in case.

- ◆ Start slow. Build up your endurance as quickly as you can without overdoing it. If you're new to exercise, you, need some time and patience to acclimate.

- ◆ Wear comfortable shoes and clothing. Blisters will sideline you, and they aren't fun.

- ◆ If you glow rather than full-out drip sweat, you may not need a shower after exercise. On the other hand, if you do sweat, you need to make plans for a shower afterward. (Most of us need showers or else we need to spend the rest of the day in isolation!)

- ◆ Beware of fitness club January specials unless you actually use the club year round. Be sure to check out your financial commitment before you sign on the dotted line.

- ◆ Plan aerobic fitness strategies for rainy days, days when you don't have a car, and days when you're on vacation or out of town. Fortunately, most hotels have fitness facilities.

◆ Exercise with a friend. This keeps both of you motivated and more likely to exercise and not skip planned sessions.

◆ Think of aerobic exercise, and any exercise for that matter, as an indulgence rather than as a chore. Everyone needs pampering and a way to let off steam. Although exercise is really a requirement, think of it as a luxury. That way, you're more likely to indulge.

◆ Keep your body hydrated. Bring along packets of Emergen-C along with bottled water. Use if and when you need to replenish your electrolytes.

◆ When you feel like you're going to boil over with stress, let off some steam through aerobic exercise.

◆ Regardless of whether you want to exercise or not, get dressed and show up. Then participate even if you can't give it your all that particular day. Failing to show up means that you could eventually give up, and you don't want to do that.

Wrong Weigh

Buyer beware of infomercial exercise products. Some work. Some don't. If you make a purchase, be sure you can return the product if you're not satisfied with your results. Also beware: You simply can't get satisfying aerobic, strength, flexibility, and health results in a couple minutes a day. So avoid gadgets that tout fitness in mere minutes a day.

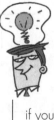

Thin-spiration

If you have the time to watch even one television show a day, you have time to exercise. Place your stationary bike in the TV room if you need to.

◆ Stretch before or after aerobic conditioning—or both. See Chapter 28 for more on stretching. Stretching keeps your muscles flexible and reduces your risk of injury.

◆ Get to know your body—its capabilities and its limits. That way, you'll be doing the best aerobic training that meets your body's needs.

◆ If something in your body starts hurting, stop exercising. Find out what's wrong and correct it before you start up again.

◆ When you start out, don't give in to your competitive urges. Instead, work at your own pace until you're ready to show off. Be sure to exercise within your heart rate range.

As you continue your aerobic conditioning, you'll discover new things about yourself and your inner strength. You'll leave the naysayers behind and establish a reliable conditioning program for yourself.

Adaptation and Progress

As you continue to exercise, your body will become accustomed to the amount and intensity of your aerobic conditioning. In other words, your aerobic exercise will become easy. This is good because you've achieved a new level of fitness. But it also means that your body is ready for more.

It's time to up the intensity or length of your workout, or both. If you're using a stationary bike, increase the resistance, pedal faster, or pedal for an additional five minutes. If you're swimming, go faster. Hike up steeper hills or take longer hikes. If you're walking, go faster or move up to speed walking. Increase the incline on your treadmill. Your body wants you to do this, so give your body exactly what it wants.

Aerobic conditioning actually pays you. Over time, you'll be paid with less fat, no insulin resistance, a stronger heart, and lower stress levels. All you need is to "just do it."

The Least You Need to Know

- Aerobic exercise increases the cells' uptake of glucose and reduces insulin resistance.

- Your body requires at least twenty minutes of aerobic exercise three times a week, and more is better.

- Aerobic exercise burns fat and elevates your mood.

- Find aerobic exercise that you enjoy and can do in a wide variety of circumstances.

Chapter

27

Boost Metabolism with Strength Training

In This Chapter

- Boosting your metabolism
- Lowering your body fat percentage
- Learning how to train for strength
- Focusing on each movement

What have you always wanted your body to look like? Certainly you want your body to be at its ideal size and to stay at that size for life. But beyond size and weight, how do you want your body to look?

Imagine yourself in a swimsuit at the beach. Most likely you want your muscles to be long and lean and toned. Certainly you want your upper arms to appear toned and tight rather than wobbly and wiggly. You can't achieve these things through what you eat, although what you eat definitely helps. You can only achieve a body that approximates your ideal through strength training.

In this chapter, you learn the very real advantages of strength training to boost your metabolism, help you lose weight, and keep it off. Plus you learn how to make your muscles strong and buff.

Benefits of Strength Training

Strength training, also known as resistance training, gives your muscles shape and definition. It also gives you many weight-loss benefits.

Avoid Weight-Loss Sagging

A very real and significant concern when losing weight is the end result. In other words, how you'll look. You could end up with sags and bags, or you could end up lean and buff. If your body shrinks in size as you lose weight without the skin area also "shrinking," you could end up with loose skin hanging around your upper arms, waist, stomach, and other areas. By the time you attain your ideal size, the only solution for tightening up your skin is plastic surgery. Plastic surgery basically cuts away the excess skin and the edges are sewn together. This is uncomfortable, expensive, and leaves you with scars. This kind of drastic situation usually only occurs when a person has more than 100 pounds to lose. But even if you have less weight to lose, you could end up with sagging skin and skin folds.

The good news is that you can avoid sagging skin by starting to do something about it today. Start strength training now and continue throughout your glycemic index weight-loss program and beyond as you maintain your new size. That way, your skin will shrink along with the rest of you. By the time you attain your ideal size, new people you meet will have no idea that you were ever overweight. Why? Because your skin will fit your body.

Strength Training and Metabolic Resistance

You've already read about metabolic resistance. It's a term used to indicate that a person's body is resistant to weight loss. Having a high percentage of body fat is the major reason for metabolic resistance.

The basic rule of metabolic activity is this: The higher a person's body fat, the slower his or her metabolism, and the harder it is to lose weight. The lower a person's body fat, the higher his or her metabolism, and the easier it is to lose weight and to maintain it.

One of the fastest ways to reduce your body fat percentage, and metabolic resistance, is with strength training. You'll love the fast results you'll achieve.

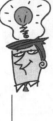

> **Thin-spiration** _____
>
> Judy's body fat was 38 percent and it seemed that no matter how much she ate or what she ate, she couldn't lose weight and keep it off. Then she started attending two one-hour Pilates classes a week. Pilates is a form of strength training. Within six months, her body fat was down to 28 percent and she was losing weight with less effort. Plus she was wearing a smaller size and her muscles looked more toned and solid.

Here's a rundown on what affects metabolism:

♦ **Age.** The younger a person, the higher his or her metabolism. As people age, their bodies need less food. Their body's hormone production slows, and the body stores more fat.

♦ **Hormones.** The lower a person's hormonal production, the lower the metabolic rate.

♦ **Body fat.** A person with high body fat has a slower metabolism.

♦ **Eating high-glycemic carbohydrates.** This can eventually lower your metabolic rate. Eating low-glycemic and higher-fiber carbohydrates can increase your metabolism.

♦ **All forms of exercise.** Exercise can increase your metabolic rate. The amount of time invested and the intensity of the exercise influences how much your metabolism is increased. But if you overdo the exercise, your metabolism can slow. So do enough, but don't overdo it.

> **Wrong Weigh** _____
>
> Julia had already lost 30 pounds, but still had 40 pounds to go. She attributed her weight loss to eating low-glycemic foods and getting plenty of exercise. When her body hit a plateau, she increased the duration and intensity of her workouts at the recommendation of her trainer. Pretty soon, she was spending two to three hours a day at the fitness center and was still on a weight-loss plateau. Julia was overtraining. By cutting back her exercise routine to about one hour a day, her body can get back in balance and start releasing stored fat again.

Obviously there's nothing you can do about your age. And although some research shows you can boost hormone production through exercise and activity, as far as anyone knows to date, you can't really turn back the hormonal clock; you can only delay its progress.

However, you can make changes with regard to your body fat and your eating. As you begin to master eating low-glycemic carbohydrates, the next step is to master your body fat percentage.

Getting Thinner, Weighing More

To understand how body fat percentage works, you need to understand that your body is comprised of three things: fat, muscle, and water. A person's water percentage ranges between about 50 percent to 60 percent. The rest is comprised of muscle or fat. It's the balance between muscle and fat that determines the portion of your weight that you have healthy control over.

Here's a chart that shows the recommended body fat percentage range for men and women by age.

Women:

Up to age 20	14% to 21%
Age 20 to 50	17% to 27%
Age 50+	20% to 30%

Men:

Up to age 20	9% to 15%
Age 20 to 50	14% to 21%
Age 50+	19% to 23%

If your body fat percentage is within the range for your age, you won't be flabby. In fact, you won't be overweight. But you could actually weigh more than you would think.

Two people who appear to be the same size and height could have very different weights. The person with a higher muscle mass will weigh more because muscle weighs more than fat. For example, suppose a woman who is 5'5" wants to weigh 125 pounds and wear a size 8. If she increases her muscle mass through strength training while she's losing weight on a glycemic index eating plan, she could get down to her desired size 8 and weigh 135 or even 140. But there's no reason for her to panic. She's wearing the size she wants to wear. Her body measurements are what she wanted. Her muscles look great—so what if she weighs more than her original goal?

Wrong Weigh

Lean people tend to have a higher percentage of water in their bodies; people who are overweight have a lower water percentage, which means they could be continually dehydrated. This can actually prevent weight loss. Be sure you're drinking at least eight glasses of water every day. Also, to help keep your body's water percentage high, you may want to supplement with electrolytes. Avoid drinking commercial electrolyte beverages that contain high-fructose corn syrup and other high-glycemic sweeteners, as well as those sweetened with artificial sweeteners. Instead, take electrolyte tablets or use a powdered drink mix such as Emergen-C.

This could happen to you, too, as you do strength training. What you weigh is less important than the size of your body. The entire situation is healthy, provided that your body fat doesn't drop below the minimum in the previous charts.

That's why it's important to set body fat percentage goals and clothing size goals as well as weight goals. Body fat percentage and clothing size are far more important than your weight goals because they're what truly tell you how you look and give you a better indication of your overall health.

Stamina, Energy, and Strength Training

Muscle gives you a performance advantage. Muscles give you stamina and endurance—not just for exercise, but for all your activities. More muscle gives you the ability to keep going when the going gets tough. You'll have more energy to do the activities you love, more energy to keep up with your children, and more ability to stay on your glycemic index weight-loss program.

Thin-spiration

As you increase your muscle mass, you may desire to go beyond the goal of increasing metabolism along with basic toning and shaping. You might decide to take up muscle building as a hobby and intentionally bulk up. In that case, you need to train longer and harder with increasingly more resistance, and you should definitely seek personal instruction.

Look Smaller Now

You want quick results, and you can achieve them with strength training. After only three months of two hour-long strength-training sessions a week, your body will become smaller. Your waist will be smaller, as will your upper arms, and your stomach will be flatter.

It will seem like everything pulls in closer to your bones, because muscle takes less space than fat. Combining glycemic index weight loss with strength training is a sure-fire way to lose weight and look smaller within weeks.

Getting Started

You only need to do two sessions of strength training a week. If you feel really ambitious, you can do three, but don't do any more than that. Strength training causes small tears in the fibers of your muscles. This is good, because as the muscles repair on your "off" days, they become stronger and tighter. If you do strength training every day, your muscles won't have time to rebuild in between sessions.

Schedule each session for 45 minutes to an hour long. Here are some equipment choices you can use for strength-training exercises:

- **Free weights.** Very popular, easy to use, widely available. Start with two- to three-pound weights and add weight as your body adapts to the weight. You'll know when this happens because the exercises will become too easy.

- **Stretch tubing.** A stretchy thin tube with handles on each end. Resembles a jump rope. You can purchase them in several levels of resistance—green, blue, red, and black.

- **Flex band.** A long, wide, stretchy band used for resistance training.

- **Ankle and wrist weights.** Strap them on for resistance as you do strengthening exercises. Don't run or jog with ankle or wrist weights, because you could overly stress your muscles and joints.

- **Body bar.** A long, weighted bar used for resistance training. May or may not have additional removable weights on either end.

- **Fitball.** A big inflated ball on which to do exercises. Seems innocent enough, but provides really challenging strength-training exercise.

◆ **Magic circle.** A circular handheld ring, about 15 inches in diameter with handles across from each other. By compressing the circle with legs, arms, and other body parts, you can get quite a workout.

◆ **Pilates classes and equipment.** An exercise method that creates long, lean, and strong muscles, plus very strong abs and terrific posture.

◆ **Exercise machines.** Those found at fitness centers. You can set the resistance of the machines to match your strength levels. They can also be purchased for home use.

◆ **Power-pump classes.** An exercise class where you lift weights and move to the beat. Fun, and the energy of the group makes the time seem to pass quickly.

There are many variations of each type of equipment and exercise. As you can see, you have plenty of choices for developing your own strength-training program.

Your First Step

Before you start using any type of equipment or strength-training system, you absolutely must learn how to do the exercises. None of them are intuitively obvious to an uneducated beginner.

If you do a strength-training exercise incorrectly, the least that could happen is that you waste your time and energy. The worst ... well ... the worst ranges from minor to major injury. Somewhere in between is bulking up the wrong muscle.

Before you start, learn the correct moves:

◆ Read an instructional book or manual. Plenty are available at bookstores and anywhere exercise equipment is sold.

◆ Take some classes. Learn the correct movements from an instructor. You need to know such things as the proper plane of movement, the proper range of movement, the speed of movement, what muscle is being worked, and how many reps are required to achieve your goal.

Thin-spiration

Not all strength-training approaches work for everyone. If you dread picking up free weights, a Pilates class may be exactly the right approach for you. You can also vary your form of strength training. You could do free weights one day and later in the week attend a power-pump class or a Pilates session.

◆ Work with a personal trainer who will give you one-on-one instruction. Most fitness centers offer personal training.

◆ Take Pilates, Fitball, and other strength-training classes, either with a group or in a private one-on-one session.

◆ Learn from exercise videos. They're inexpensive and at-home convenient. Collagevideo.com stocks hundreds of titles, and they sell some equipment, such as Fitballs, stretch tubing, body bars, and flex bands.

You'll have fun and get results even as you learn how to do strength training.

Thin-spiration

A new method of weight training recommends doing very slow repetitions of each exercise, so that a person can't use any momentum in the movement. Momentum definitely makes a move easier. Find out whether this approach will work well for you by trying it. Overall, going slowly can be highly effective. You do fewer repetitions of each exercise, but take longer with each one.

Mindfulness

Unlike aerobic conditioning, where your mind can wander off while you huff and puff, strength training requires that you also engage your mind at the same time that you engage your muscles. The more you can mentally focus on each movement as opposed to doing mindless reps, the more successful your efforts will be.

Concentration is key to your success. In fact, as you're doing the exercises, you may find yourself wishing that you could simply bliss out. But don't. Letting your mind wander can lead to injury.

Many people find strength training to be a form of meditation and relaxation because they can't dwell on their day-to-day concerns during a session.

Around the Middle

Losing inches from your waist and abdomen area is excellent for your physique and also great for your health. People who have high fat distribution around the midsection are more likely to develop chronic and life-threatening health conditions. These include heart disease, diabetes, metabolic resistance, metabolic syndrome, high blood pressure, and even cancers.

You've already chosen to use glycemic index weight loss as a way to trim fat from your midsection. Use strength training as well.

Be sure that you do the following kinds of exercises and techniques to trim your entire midsection, known as your core:

◆ Good old-fashioned abdominal crunches are still the best basic exercise for your midsection. Make sure that you pull your navel into your spine as you do each crunch. Don't let your stomach pooch out as you do crunches because this will strengthen muscles that give you a potbelly.

◆ Whenever you do an exercise that requires stomach strength, think "navel to spine" and pull in your stomach.

◆ Do abdominal crunches, sit-ups, and roll-ups in which you work your waist and transverse abdominal muscles. One such exercise would be partial sit-ups done with your hands behind your head. As you sit up, touch your elbow to the opposite knee. These are tough, but very effective for toning the waist and abs.

◆ Do crunches and roll-ups on the Fitball. Ouch. The curve of the ball and the need for core stability as you do a crunch work the full range of your abdominal muscle group.

◆ Take a core-conditioning class to learn other exercises that strengthen and tone your core.

In the next chapter, you learn stretches that also keep your midsection, as well as your entire body, thin and toned.

The Least You Need to Know

◆ Strength training boosts your metabolism and reduces metabolic resistance to weight loss.

◆ Strength training quickly reduces body-fat percentage and increases muscle mass.

◆ Before you start a strength-training program, learn the correct way to do each exercise.

◆ Use strength training to keep your waist, midriff, and abdominal areas toned and trim.

Chapter 28

Stretching for Weight Loss

In This Chapter

◆ Stretching your way to weight loss

◆ Reducing cortisol levels and easing aches and pains

◆ Learning how to stretch

◆ Stretching to tone your midsection

Cats, dogs, and other animals do it. We're not so sure about the birds and the bees, but we know for certain that only some people do it. Which is too bad, because everyone can benefit from doing it regularly.

Yes, we're talking about stretching. Until recently, stretching was thought of as an exercise-program add-on. Exercise experts agreed that stretching was a good practice for staying limber and reducing injury, but fitness centers didn't offer stretching classes. At best, it was recommended that a person stretch for five minutes before or after aerobic exercise. What a loss.

Stretching is the third and final aspect of a complete exercise routine. In this chapter, you learn how stretching enhances your glycemic index weight-loss efforts and you learn the long and short of flexible-muscle maintenance.

Stretching Connection

It's not immediately obvious that there's a connection between stretching and weight loss. You don't burn more calories when you stretch. In fact, you hardly use any energy at all. Stretching has little to do with eating, except for the fact that it's difficult to eat when stretching. Your stretching time is time away from food, but that could hardly enhance your weight-loss efforts. So just how are glycemic index weight loss and stretching connected?

The Cortisol Connection

In previous chapters, we discussed that when your stress level rises, so does your body's level of the hormone insulin. This leads to insulin resistance and, ultimately, weight gain. So keeping your stress levels low also benefits weight loss.

Now here's how stretching fits into this cortisol/insulin situation. When you're stressed, your muscles tighten. You've probably noticed that your shoulders seem to turn into solid knots as you work frantically on your keyboard to meet a deadline.

You may also be familiar with tension headaches. A stressful situation prompts you to get tense, your muscles tighten, and before long you have a tension headache, a backache, or a leg cramp. We all carry stress in our muscles.

You must remove the stress from your muscles to release it. Stretching does just that. Many people have found that the secret to relieving headaches and backaches isn't found in the medicine cabinet or with a professional massage, but rather in taking five to ten minutes or more to stretch.

Stretching removes muscular tensions, lightens stress loads, and reduces cortisol levels, making it easier to lose weight.

Muscle Strain

Any time you use your muscles in new ways, a situation is created that causes a buildup of muscular tension and tightness. Activities that can cause muscular tension include strength training, sprains, aerobic exercise, anger, fear, anxiety, accidents, surgeries, illness, and even allergies. Even toting a heavy carry-on bag through the airport can leave shoulders, arms, and even fingers tense, creating muscle aches and tightness.

The first reason this is a problem is that the tension makes your muscles hurt and the aches can last for days. The second reason is that the same aching muscles increase your cortisol levels. How can you solve both problems? You guessed it—stretch out those muscles. Not only will you lower your cortisol levels, you may also find that the actual situation that caused the tension improves.

The bottom line here is this: Muscle tension of any kind increases cortisol levels. Stretching releases muscle tension, lowers cortisol levels, and speeds up healing.

Stretching as Detox

When you stretch your muscles, you're helping to release toxins that are stored in fat and muscle. Stretching also helps move the lymph fluid that removes toxins through the body. Because toxin buildup can thwart weight loss, removing those toxins by stretching can further assist your glycemic index weight-loss efforts. See Chapter 25 for more information on how toxins are stored in fat.

Aches and Pains

If you've dealt with serious aches and pains in your life, such as chronic back pain, you know how easily this gets in the way of losing weight. Even if you eat correctly, the pain can be a barrier against getting to your ideal size. It makes exercise unappealing, because it can be painful—at least at first.

Many doctors and physical therapists now use combination therapies to reduce pain. They continue to prescribe medicines and massage, but they also recommend stretching exercises to help reduce chronic pain and the stress caused by the pain, as well as to increase the range of movement. Again, the bottom line is this: Less pain means less stress, which results in lowered cortisol levels, which lowers insulin levels, which promotes weight loss.

Thin-spiration

Joe was 45 when he began a stretching routine. He enjoyed racquetball and fencing, but found that he had trouble walking down steps the following mornings. His body was stiff and sore. His first five or ten stretching classes seemed brutal, as he was releasing athletic tensions and muscle bulk built up over the years. Within a couple of months, he noticed the stretching was easier and he was trading bulk and heft for a more graceful, yet strong body. His new muscle agility reduced his "morning-after racquetball" aches and pains.

Day-to-Day Stress

If your life is basically in balance, you're probably experiencing only normal, everyday stress. Still, stretching can assist you in regulating your cortisol levels and easing your way to weight loss. Use stretching to soothe your moods, refresh your body, and work out the kinks that result from normal daily activities and your exercise program.

Preventing Injuries

Traditionally, stretching has been recommended by exercise specialists as a way to reduce the likelihood of sports-related and exercise-related injuries. Flexible athletes can better withstand the bodily assaults they experience from contact sports and repetitive movements. In fact, many professional athletes now participate in yoga and Pilates classes as a way to keep their muscles stretched, agile, and flexible.

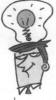

Thin-spiration

Practically speaking, agility is important for regular living. You want to have the agility that enables you to easily bend over, climb steps, and do basic everyday movements, such as tying your shoes and unloading the dishwasher. You need agility for all sorts of simple movements, not to mention being able to enjoy getting out on the dance floor and kicking up your heels.

Most likely, you aren't a professional athlete, but you can use stretching to receive the same benefits. Now that you're doing regular aerobic exercise and strength training, you need stretching to continue your fitness training comfortably for years to come. You also need to stay flexible so that you can benefit from the weight-loss and weight-maintenance benefits of aerobic exercise and strength training.

The Illusion of Slim

Having a longer and elongated body through stretching makes you appear slimmer as you lose weight. Your clothes will fit better and your posture will improve. Looking better and feeling better about the way you look reinforces your glycemic index weight-loss efforts.

Getting Started

You are already a "natural" for stretching. You don't need to have lots of skill, but simply desire and some time. You don't need any equipment, but the following can be helpful:

◆ Clothing that is nonbinding and lets you move. You can wear a T-shirt and athletic-type shorts. You can also wear stretch clothing, such as a leotard and tights, or yoga pants and top.

◆ No shoes are required.

◆ A sticky mat that can be rolled up is useful, but not necessary.

Next, you need to set aside time to stretch. Plan to stretch for ten to fifteen minutes at least every other day. Again, more is better. You may find that as you begin to realize the benefits of stretching, you want to spend more time doing it.

The most important rule in stretching, whether you're a beginner or are advanced, is this: *Never overdo it.* Don't try to stretch farther than your muscles can comfortably release. When you stretch a muscle, your body sends you clear signals regarding how much is enough. It's painful to overdo it, and you could pull a muscle.

You could also pull a muscle if you aren't warmed up before you stretch. Exercise physiologists recommend warming up for two to five minutes before you begin stretching. This increases circulation and body heat, which makes your muscles stretch easier. Warm-up activities include walking, climbing stairs, and jogging.

For successful and effective stretching, follow this simple advice. Go slow to go fast. Take your time and pretty soon you, too, will be putting your hands on the floor when you bend over to touch your toes. All it takes is patience, tenacity, and perseverance. If your muscles hurt, then back off and only stretch as far as you are comfortable.

When you see a person who seems highly flexible, ask how long it took them to get to that level. Some people are simply born flexible, but most people need to work at it. If you've never stretched before in your life, expect to find it challenging to stretch and attain body flexibility. But don't give up. The results are well worth it.

> **Thin-spiration**
>
> Even though stretching is easiest in loose-fitting clothing, don't let the wrong attire prevent you from stretching at your desk or on the floor of your office during a break. You may want to keep a yoga-type sticky mat in your office for stretch breaks.

> **Wrong Weigh**
>
> Be sure to hold each stretch when you reach your maximum stretch position. Don't bounce, but rather hold the position for twenty seconds to two minutes. As you do this, the muscles release and tensions melt away.

Where and When to Stretch

You can stretch almost anywhere that you have some space and relative privacy. Good locations and times for stretching include the following:

◆ At your desk. You'll be amazed at how many stretches you can do while seated in your chair.

◆ On the floor of your office. Use a mat or towel.

◆ Before and after aerobic exercise. Keeps your calves, hamstrings, and Achilles tendon flexible and supple.

◆ After strength training. Helps pull from your muscles the buildup of lactic acid that can cause soreness the next day. If you're sore the next day, stretch again.

◆ While watching television. Get down on the floor and stretch during your favorite shows.

◆ While in the kitchen preparing meals. Usually the kitchen counter is just the right height for leg extension stretches (like ballerinas would do at the barre).

◆ At fitness classes, such as yoga and Pilates mat classes.

◆ After long periods spent sitting, as in car trips, airplane travel, or seminars.

◆ First thing in the morning when you get out of bed or after your morning shower. Especially great if you're dealing with chronic aches and pains.

◆ When you get home from work as a way to decompress and relax.

Stretching is flexible, no pun intended. You can stretch virtually anywhere and relish the benefits wherever you happen to be.

Learning How to Stretch

Stretching is a very safe and comfortable activity, but even so, you need to learn which muscles to stretch and how. Use one or more of the following tools to learn:

◆ An instructor, such as a yoga teacher, physical therapist, Pilates instructor, or fitness trainer.

◆ A book. One classic book that's been used for more than 25 years is *Stretching*, by Bob Anderson. You can find it at bookstores or online.

◆ Exercise videos and DVDs. These offer at-home learning. A good selection of offerings can be found at collagevideo.com.

◆ Take several basic stretching fitness classes. Unfortunately, you can't always rely on yoga classes to teach you the basics of stretching. Some are too exotic or unbalanced in their approach.

After you learn the basics of stretching your basic muscle groups, there is still more to learn. But you should first learn how to stretch your basic major muscle groups before moving on to advanced stretching.

Stretching Methods

As you delve into stretching, you'll find several different methods and systems. Because stretching is as ancient as humankind, and because you have only a limited number of muscles that can be stretched, the systems are fundamentally the same. You can choose from any of the methods listed here:

◆ Yoga is an ancient system for stretching and well-being. Hatha yoga, the yoga of body movement, has many branches, such as Iyengar, Bikram, Astanga, and others. If you're just starting out, take a class that works with the basics. You can explore the other forms in depth later if you're so inclined. The yoga offered at most fitness centers is basic Hatha yoga.

◆ All-American stretching, as explained in the book *Stretching*, by Bob Anderson.

◆ Pilates is a recent exercise form that incorporates core strengthening with muscle toning and superb stretching. In one class you do both strength training and stretching. Pilates builds long, lean muscles and corrects any postural misalignments. You'll even stand up straighter.

◆ You can use equipment in your stretching that can intensify the stretch and enhance your workout. Such equipment includes flex bands, stretch tubing, and Fitballs.

> **Thin-spiration**
>
> If you're frustrated because you can't seem to lose weight and your muscles are strong and bulky, use this approach: Cut back on your strength training and increase the time you spend stretching. The stretching will help elongate muscles and reduce bulk, thus enhancing your weight-loss momentum. Alternate aerobics and strength training days, and stretch every day.

Be sure to include stretching when you put together your master exercise program. All three aspects of exercise—aerobic conditioning, strength training, and stretching—work synergistically to give you the shape, stamina, and health you desire.

Stretching for a Flatter Tummy

Stretching is also a great tool to minimize your midsection. You'll love the results. Here arc some stretches to use:

◆ Do reverse abdominal stretching after your crunches and sit-ups. Use a large Fitball and roll back over it so that you're facing the ceiling, with your hands touching the floor behind you and your feet or toes on the floor in front. This stretches your abs as well as the psoas muscles that run from the side of your abdomen down the front side of your leg.

◆ Lie over a Fitball facing the floor with your stomach on the ball. Very slowly, roll on the ball—pausing as each vertebra receives a nice stretch that opens it up. This helps elongate the spine and actually makes your midsection appear slimmer.

◆ Stretch your body laterally—that is, to the side. Target the muscles that run from the sides of your legs up through the sides of your body. Side bends are great.

Thin-spiration

To have a tight and flat abdominal area, you need to stretch your abdominal area muscles as well as strengthen them with crunches, sit-ups, and other core training exercises. Don't omit the stretching. It can reduce bulky muscles and smooth out the way your gut looks.

Remember to hold the position when you reach your maximum extension for each exercise. You can also sit on the floor with legs apart and bend over laterally to touch the toes on one foot. Hold. And then stretch to the other foot. Often, stretching- and yoga-class instructors forget about the important slimming lateral stretches.

Experiment with stretches. When you find one that especially stretches your midsection, use it over and over again to regain your youthful figure.

The Least You Need to Know

◆ Add a stretching routine to your exercise program to enhance your ability to lose weight.

◆ Stretching can help decrease the size of bulky muscles and make you look slimmer.

◆ Stretching helps reduce cortisol levels, detoxify the body, and soothe moods.

◆ Do at least two fifteen-minute stretching sessions a week, but more is better.

Part 7

Glycemic Index Books and Programs

Several excellent books contain eating programs that incorporate aspects of the glycemic index. Some of the programs are designed for weight loss and some are designed to improve your health—one is even specifically designed for women experiencing a change of life.

Learn about the best books for further exploring the scientific and nutritional basis of the glycemic index.

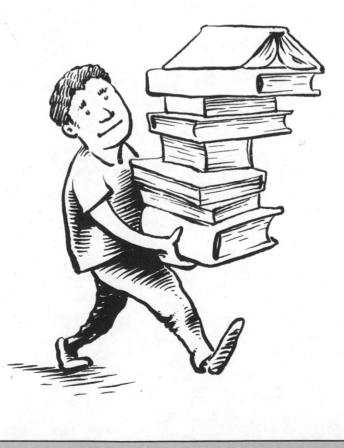

Chapter 29

Glycemic Index Resources and Support

In This Chapter

◆ Learning about weight-loss programs featuring the glycemic index

◆ Learning which programs could work for you

◆ Understanding the caveperson's diet

◆ Eating for a lifetime with the glycemic index

The number of informational and support resources available on the glycemic index is growing every day. Be assured that you'll continue to find more and more as the popularity and viability of the glycemic index grows.

Right now you are on the leading edge of a whole new way of thinking about weight loss and eating. The ground swell of the glycemic index has only begun.

In this chapter we give you information on the best resources available. As of this writing, the most popular diet systems such as Weight Watchers,

Jenny Craig, eDiets, and others don't include the glycemic index as a significant part of their eating programs. Most likely they will soon.

The New Glucose Revolution

The New Glucose Revolution was the first book to popularize eating low-glycemic foods. It was first published in 1999. The authors, Jennie Brand-Miller, Ph.D.; Thomas M. S. Wolever, M.D., Ph.D.; Kaye Foster-Powell, M. Nutr. & Diet; and Stephen Colagiuri, M.D., are well-versed in the science of carbohydrates and their effects on the body's insulin levels and blood glucose levels. They discuss the need for eating

mostly low-glycemic carbohydrates and explain how high-glycemic carbohydrates aren't good for your health or waistline.

> ### Body of Knowledge
>
> David J. A. Jenkins is credited as the first person to recognize that not all carbohydrates are created equal. He created the glycemic index while doing research on diabetes at the University of Toronto, Canada.

But, they explain, neither is eating too many low-glycemic carbohydrates. Their point is that the glycemic index of a particular carbohydrate reveals only half the equation. The other half is the glycemic load, which, as you know, mathematically takes into account the glycemic index of a food *and* the quantity eaten.

The New Glucose Revolution Features

The authors recommend eating about 250 grams of carbs a day. They suggest that eating low-glycemic carbs promotes health, but suggest it's fine to eat medium- and even high-glycemic carbs—provided that an average person who's not on a weight-loss program eats a glycemic load of between 138 and 163 for the day. They don't make recommendations for weight loss.

What the Program Misses

Although the book advocates eating good fats in somewhat general terms, it doesn't emphasize the important role of essential fatty acids in a person's overall health. But the authors do advocate eating a diet low in fats, which we applaud.

The authors promote eating low- and medium-glycemic starches, even for people who want to lose weight, but don't discuss the prevalence of food allergies to wheat and other starches that can promote weight gain. For a dieter, they recommend four servings of breads, pasta, cereal, rice, or noodles per day. This is too much starch for many overweight people and certainly too much for people who are metabolically resistant to weight loss.

Hits the Mark

We sincerely thank the authors for their research on the glycemic index. Without their efforts and courage, we might never have been able to understand the biology of insulin resistance and the effects that carbohydrates have on weight gain and weight management.

The book was not written as a book on weight loss, but rather as a guide to healthy eating. The back of the book contains an extensive list of many carbohydrate foods, giving their glycemic index along with their glycemic load. The list includes many brand name foods, including cereals and baked goods.

This book became the springboard for a series of companion books by the same authors. One of them, *What Makes My Blood Glucose Go Up … and Down?*, is discussed next.

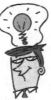

Thin-spiration

We can only hope that all food manufacturers soon include the glycemic index and glycemic load on their product nutritional analysis labels. This information would be tremendously helpful when shopping for food. It would give you a better idea of how a packaged food would affect your blood sugar levels and how much it would stimulate insulin production.

What Makes My Blood Glucose Go Up … and Down?

What Makes My Blood Glucose Go Up … and Down? by Jennie Brand-Miller, Ph.D.; Kay Foster-Powell, M. Nutr. & Diet; and Rick Mendosa answers 101 frequently asked questions about blood glucose levels. The book is written primarily for persons with diabetes, but we've found it to be an excellent guide for eating based on the glycemic index.

As you read through this book, remember that when your blood glucose, also known as blood

Thin-spiration

Don't miss the glycemic index listing at the back of the book, *What Makes My Blood Glucose Go Up … and Down?* It has updated values for many carbohydrates that have been misunderstood in earlier lists, namely carrots, dates, yams, peaches, and others.

sugar, levels are stable and low, so are your insulin levels. This situation helps you continue to lose weight, avoid more fat storage, and avoid the possibility of having metabolic syndrome.

This book isn't a weight-loss guide and doesn't offer a program, but it can guide you to a better understanding of your body and its needs for low-glycemic carbohydrates.

The GI Diet

The GI Diet was originally published in Canada, where it's been highly successful. The book's popularity has since spread to the United States. The author, Rick Gallop, offers a simple plan of low-glycemic eating combined with good fats and lean meats.

The GI Diet Features

You won't find yourself counting or calculating in this plan; instead, you eat foods based on whether they're listed in the red, yellow, or green lists. Red foods are foods you should avoid or eat very infrequently. Yellow foods are marginally acceptable, but you won't eat much of them. By contrast, green foods are a "go." Eat them in moderate amounts and you'll lose weight and feel better.

You'll do plenty of healthful exercise by following the exercise guidelines and tracking your progress with the exercise diary forms. Plus resistance training is included, which is great for everyone, but is especially advantageous for a person who's metabolically resistant to weight loss.

CAUTION

Wrong Weigh

We urge you to avoid artificial sweeteners, even though Gallop gives them the green light in *The GI Diet*. At the very least, they stimulate appetite. But some research shows they can also lead to metabolic and health disorders. Because the use of artificial sweeteners such as aspartame and sucralose is controversial, your best bet is to avoid them altogether.

What the Program Misses

The GI Diet is a simple solution that doesn't address such issues as stress hormones, the body burden of toxins, and emotional eating. Still, even without these, anyone can follow this color-cued approach.

More significantly, the book doesn't address glycemic load at all, but instead gives you recommended serving sizes. If you use this program, be sure to carefully follow the program so that you don't overeat or eat too high a glycemic load.

The diet recommends limiting fats more than you need to. It really is okay to eat whole eggs in moderate amounts, but the diet puts regular whole eggs in the red zone. It also supports the use of artificial sweeteners that are known to stimulate appetite and whose safety is highly controversial.

Hits the Mark

If you want a very simple low-glycemic weight-loss program, this one can work well. The program is nutritionally sound, but extreme in strictly limiting fat. In fact, you'll lose weight on this program even if you ease up on the fat restrictions. Although it's true that too much overall fat can cause insulin resistance, what works best for weight control and decreasing insulin resistance is to eat about 20 percent to 30 percent of total calories from fat.

The Zone

Although *The Zone* is considered by many people to be a low-carb program, it actually recommends eating low-glycemic carbohydrates. Barry Sears, the author, suggests that an ideally balanced diet is 30 percent protein, 30 percent fat, and 40 percent carbs, which can work for many people.

The Zone advocates eating lean meats, good fats, and low-glycemic carbohydrates. You'll be eating plenty of vegetables and fruits, so you're certain to eat at least 5, and more like 10, servings a day.

When *The Zone* was originally published, the concept that high-glycemic carbohydrates cause insulin-resistance was new information. So was the distinction between good and bad fats.

The Zone is a good weight-loss program and can assist you in eating based on the glycemic index.

The Paleo Diet

Loren Cordaine used the point of view of evolutionary biology in developing his eating program. The premise is this: Human DNA today is virtually identical to cavemen and cavewomen. The foods they ate for more than seven million years are the same foods that our bodies are still best adapted to digest and assimilate. And surprise, those foods are definitely low-glycemic. All around, The Paleo Diet is a winner.

Body of Knowledge

Okay, it's true. Most of our prehistoric ancestors didn't actually live in caves; they tended to live in more open environments. But you get the point. Our bodies are virtually identical genetically to our oldest human forebears. Although our wonderful brains have made it possible for us to further develop agriculture and advanced cuisine—if Jello can be considered advanced—our bodies still work much like the bodies of our prehistoric ancestors.

Cordaine's major premise is that our bodies are not as well suited to digest and assimilate foods that have only recently been introduced into the human diet. Makes sense so far. Now here's what's so surprising.

It's only been during the past 10,000 years that humans have eaten grains and dairy foods. That may seem like a long time, but 10,000 years is just a tick-tock of the clock compared to the previous seven million years of human evolution. Cordaine points out that many people have allergic reactions or food sensitivities to grains and dairy. But that's not all. Coffee, tea, refined sugar, enriched flour, artificial sweeteners, and chemical preservatives are even newer in the human diet and we are less suited to consuming them, too.

By eating a Paleo Diet, Cordaine claims people can lose weight easily, maintain the weight loss, and stay healthier.

The Paleo Diet Features

Caveperson foods are meats, fish, poultry, eggs, vegetables and fruits, nuts and seeds, and some honey. According to Cordaine, these foods contain all the nutrition anyone needed in the past or now. This only makes sense. If our ancient ancestors weren't able to obtain necessary nutrients from their foods, the human race would have died out millions of years ago.

Cordaine recommends that you avoid eating modern foods, such as foods made from grains including cereals, muffins, cookies, pancakes, and such. He also recommends that you avoid eating dairy products.

On the Paleo Diet, you won't eat starches, dairy, refined sugars, or sodas. Which means your carbohydrate intake will limit itself naturally to low-glycemic foods. If you take away the carbohydrates introduced into the human diet within the past

10,000 years, the only carbs left are vegetables, fruits, nuts, seeds, and honey. They're basically all low-glycemic. (The glycemic index for honey ranges widely, but some honeys are low-glycemic.)

The program isn't strict, but it certainly can be called restrictive. And yes, you can cheat. Some. For instance, the author admits to a fondness for wine, and we're sure you could figure out how to eat some chocolate and still be 90 percent faithful to eating like your "inner caveperson." The book advocates getting plenty of hearty exercise just as our ancient ancestors did daily.

What the Program Misses

The Paleo Diet doesn't miss. The science is solid and the program quite simply works. Cordaine covers glycemic index, glycemic load, and the need to avoid overeating.

It's unrealistic to think that many people could easily give up the all-enticing nuances of modern day foods and revert to primitive eating, but we find the information helpful in understanding our genetics and the basics of healthy eating.

Hits the Mark

The program is so simple that anyone can understand it. There's no weighing and no measuring. You don't even need to count. You might find it tricky to eat at a Mexican food restaurant, but then, you would also find it tricky to eat at a Mexican-food restaurant based on any glycemic index weight-loss program.

If you are plagued with allergies, candida, high-blood pressure, heart disease, diabetes, fatigue, mood disorders, autoimmune diseases, or other chronic health problems, give the Paleo Diet a try and eat as a caveperson would for a month or two. You might be amazed with your results and with your weight loss. The recommended foods don't trigger cortisol release, so they can help lighten your stress load and emotional eating patterns.

The Fat Flush Plan

The Fat Flush Plan offers you everything you need—including up-to-date science—to detoxify your body and feel great while reaching your ideal size. The author, Ann Louise Gittleman, is concerned about a person's total health, including emotional well-being. She presents a totally comprehensive plan that includes all aspects of lifestyle as it relates to weight gain and weight loss. You'll find information about ways to eat low-glycemic while enjoying good fats and lean meats. Plus, it includes a specific exercise program, ways to combat stress-related weight gain, and a method to detoxify your body so that your body can flush out the fat from your hips, waist, and thighs.

The Fat Flush Plan Features

In Gittleman's book, you'll find biological and nutritional explanations of all the elements of the program. You'll learn how the liver removes toxins from the body and how it functions to release stored fat. The explanations are clear and useful.

The program is integrated into every area of your life, from what you do upon rising in the morning to going to sleep at night. In between those times, you do detoxifying physical exercises, drink cranberry and long-life cocktails, and journal.

The program has three phases, which include a two-week fat-flush phase, an ongoing fat-flush phase, and a third phase called the Lifestyle Eating Plan.

You learn how to eat while traveling, how to shop for groceries, and, essentially, how to live the fat-flush way.

What the Program Misses

We can't think of a thing wrong from a health point of view. However, compliance with this eating plan requires high commitment and mindfulness.

Thin-spiration

The Fat Flush Plan appeals specifically to middle-aged women who are wrestling with weight gain due to hormonal imbalances. The author understands this frustration and many women in their 40s, 50s, and 60s have experienced success with this program.

Hits the Mark

If you want a totally comprehensive, low-glycemic lifestyle program, this one's for you. The program is very specific, so be prepared to eat the recommended foods and to follow the program carefully. Doing the program comprehensively takes time and planning, but you'll appreciate the results.

This program works well if you're metabolically resistant to weight loss or have midlife hormonal concerns. If you know that you've been exposed to heavy doses of environmental toxins that could be affecting your health or your life, give the Fat Flush Plan a try. Also consider using this program if you have weight gain specifically around your midsection.

The Perricone Prescription

Yes, *The Perricone Prescription* is a book about skin care, so why are we reviewing it? Because Dr. Nicholas Perricone offers a low-glycemic diet designed to improve the condition of your skin, and, coincidentally, it's a superb weight-loss diet. Amazing.

His theory is that eating low-glycemic foods along with good fats reduces inflammation. Inflammation causes undesirable skin conditions such as sagging, wrinkles, acne, and congestion. He shows how the cause of the inflammation is increased insulin levels. Yes, the same insulin levels you are managing by eating the glycemic index way.

Perricone gives you a menu to follow for the first 14 days. You then repeat the menu for another 14 days and you'll have completed your first 28 days of creating better skin, but you'll also be losing weight. The book includes recipes that help you manage your insulin levels and help you eat plenty of healthy protein, good fats, and moderate amounts of low-glycemic carbs.

The Perricone Prescription also includes exercise as a top priority for skin health. Because the body is a total reflection of a person's general state of health, what a person does through diet and exercise to improve the skin also benefits the whole body and vice versa. After 28 days, you'll have better skin, and you'll also have a smaller body.

You can then continue to follow Dr. Perricone's eating plan to lose weight. We think you'll like the results.

Thin-spiration

If you find the very thought of weight loss to be unappealing, how about following an eating plan that improves the quality of your skin and, as a side benefit, lets you lose weight plus improve your overall health? This just could be the low-glycemic weight-loss program for you.

Dr. Atkins's New Diet Revolution

And what a revolution he created! Dr. Robert Atkins was the first to advise us to stop counting calories and, instead, to count carbohydrates. That was in the early 1970s. Needless to say, the medical and dietetic communities didn't warmly embrace his weight-loss philosophy. In fact, support for Atkins's approach has only come in recent years.

The details of the program that Dr. Atkins espoused in the 1970s are considerably different from the recommendations found in his latest book. Early on he advocated eating large amounts of meats and eggs and wasn't fond of any carbohydrates, even vegetables. Dr. Atkins's program evolved over the past 30 years as new research revealed the problems with eating saturated fats, the health benefits of eating 5 to 10 servings daily of vegetables, and the creation of the glycemic index. In fact, in his most recent books, Dr. Atkins included a glycemic index list and advised his readers to eat low-glycemic.

We're giving you some information on the Atkins approach so that you can understand the differences between his program and your glycemic index weight-loss program. We don't recommend the Atkins approach. Eating based on the glycemic index gives you excellent results without an induction phase or eating unbalanced meals.

Atkins Program Features

Today's Atkins program includes the following features:

- ◆ Begins with a two-week induction phase limiting carbs to two cups of free vegetables and one serving of other low-glycemic vegetables per day.

- ◆ Puts a person into ketosis during the induction phase.

- ◆ Adds back only five grams of carbs per day per week during the ongoing weight-loss program.

- ◆ Recommends eating low-glycemic carbs over high-glycemic carbs in the maintenance phase.

- ◆ Strongly urges the dieter to avoid caffeine and the artificial sweetener aspartame.

We now know that you don't need a three-phase program to lose weight. In fact, you don't need to go into ketosis to lose weight. And we know that your body needs more vegetables than allowed on this program.

What the Program Misses

Dr. Atkins's program gives comprehensive advice about which kinds of carbohydrates to eat and how to eat them, but it falls short in the following areas:

◆ It ignores the fact that high stress levels can cause weight gain and prevent weight loss.

◆ It doesn't consider body fat percentage as an important factor in determining a person's ease in losing weight.

◆ It doesn't recommend adding strength-training exercise sessions as a way to reduce body fat. Strength training reduces a person's metabolic resistance to weight loss. Instead, it advocates using the induction program to reduce metabolic resistance.

◆ It is too strict with free foods. These have virtually no glycemic load and they don't need to be restricted. A person isn't permitted to eat 5 to 10 servings of vegetables and fruits during the induction phase, and perhaps not even during the ongoing phase.

The Atkins program missing the mark in these areas probably explains why some dieters fail to lose weight on the program. The glycemic index weight-loss program takes all these factors into account so that you get the results you want.

The South Beach Diet

This newcomer to the weight-loss world has gained a terrific following. The cover of the book claims that you'll lose belly fat first. Who wouldn't like that? Actually, all low-glycemic weight-loss programs could make the same claim, because eating low-glycemic meals reduces the size of your waist and tummy quickly.

The South Beach Diet, written by Dr. Arthur Agatston, offers two features of great importance. The first is that it incorporates the latest research on the wisdom of eating certain foods, such as good fats, low-glycemic carbohydrates, and lean meats. Next, the maintenance phase is totally flexible, allowing you to eat high-glycemic carbs and even junk foods, provided that you don't start gaining weight.

The three-phase eating plan is great in phases one and two, but seems to get confused and doesn't continue advocating eating mostly low-glycemic carbohydrates in the maintenance phase. The well-intended premise is that by the time you reach phase three, your eating preferences are reformed, and you'll only want to eat the healthiest foods, including low-glycemic carbs. This is wishful thinking, because most dieters are longing to return to their old eating habits. But we hope we're proved wrong on this point.

Finally, the program doesn't mention glycemic load, which is an excellent tool for knowing exactly how much to eat to lose weight and to maintain your weight loss.

The Least You Need to Know

♦ Some specialty weight-loss programs are excellent for low-glycemic weight loss and for improving health.

♦ The popular skin care program of Dr. Nicholas Perricone offers an excellent low-glycemic weight-loss program.

♦ Take advantage of the excellent books and resources on glycemic index weight loss.

♦ Avoid weight-loss programs that have induction programs or which deprive you of eating balanced meals.

♦ Eating foods that harmonize with your biology can promote health, reduce allergic reactions, and increase your overall wellness.

A

Glossary

adipose tissue   Another term for body fat that you want to lose. It's a brown color and is the fat that's used for fuel when you are on a low-carb weight-loss program.

aerobic exercise   Exercise that you do for a sustained amount of time, for at least 15 minutes, that moves your major muscles and makes you huff and puff and break into a sweat. Running, jogging, swimming, and bicycling are popular forms. But vigorous hiking, racquetball, tennis, or dancing are also considered aerobic exercise, as are aerobic conditioning classes. Golf, bowling, and billiards aren't.

alkaline ash   The result of urine turning more alkaline. When the body is slightly alkaline, it's easier for it to maintain the proper bacteria-yeast balance level so that a person can reduce or eliminate urinary tract infections as well as yeast infections.

basal metabolic rate   The rate at which a person's body uses energy in a resting state, such as sitting still. The body really does "burn" through food, actually producing heat and providing energy to your organs and muscles.

blood sugar level   Your blood sugar level is considered healthy when the fasting level is between 80 and 120. This can be measured at a doctor's office.

body burden   The amount of toxins an individual has in the body at any point in time.

body fat percentage   A measurement of a person's body fat. The total amount of body fat, muscle mass, and water a person has equals 100 percent. Body fat percentage can be measured at a health center, a doctor's office, or a fitness club.

complete proteins   Foods that contain all nine essential amino acids. Proteins from meat, fish, fowl, shellfish, and dairy are complete proteins. Cheeses offer more protein per ounce than milk and yogurt.

cortisol   A stress hormone secreted by the adrenal glands that stimulates the release of glycogen stores in the liver and in the muscles. Glycogen is the body's storage form of carbohydrate that breaks down into blood glucose in times of need. The extra blood glucose produced by cortisol increases stamina, endurance, and mental acuity during times of stress. Cortisol levels are high when a person's short- or long-term stress is high. Elevated cortisol levels often lead to such chronic conditions as weight gain, diabetes, heart disease, cancer, and high blood pressure.

essential fatty acids (EFAs)   Polyunsaturated fats that are essential for your health. They can be obtained only by ingesting them, thus the government designation of "essential." The two main essential fatty acids are alpha-linolenic acid (an omega-3 fatty acid), and linoleic acid (an omega-6 fatty acid).

fruit ogliosaccharides (FOS)   A probiotic nutritional supplement that selectively nourishes the friendly bacteria in the intestines. It increases the number of good bacteria in your gut. Not only is stevia safe, FOSes are definitely good for you.

glycemic load   Measures the total impact of an amount of food on blood sugar levels. To calculate the load, multiply the number of grams of carbohydrate in a food by its glycemic index.

glyconutrients   Sugars that naturally occur in plants. Some, such as galactose (a milk sugar) and glucose, taste sweet. The others are not sweet. All are needed by the body for important metabolic processes.

high-glycemic foods   Carbohydrates that trigger a quick rise in blood sugar levels. These are such foods as bread, cookies, sodas, white potatoes, some packaged breakfast cereals, and highly refined grains. Low-glycemic foods are foods such as green vegetables, many fruits, legumes, and nuts that cause a slight and safe rise in blood sugar levels. Medium-glycemic foods include table sugar, some dried fruits, and some whole-grain crackers and breads that cause a moderate rise. In the induction phase of a low-carb weight-loss program, you eat only low-glycemic carbohydrates. See Appendix B for a listing of the glycemic index of many foods.

incomplete proteins   Foods that don't contain all nine essential amino acids. These foods are vegetables or vegetable-based, such as soybeans, nuts, legumes, and grains.

induction phase   A standard part of low-carb as opposed to low-glycemic weight-loss programs. In the two-week induction phase, a person eats strictly limited amounts of carbohydrates, most of which are "free vegetables." Induction phase eating is out-of-balance and not necessary for weight loss.

insulin resistance   A condition that occurs when the body's cells no longer readily uptake glucose for energy from insulin. The cells are then, in a sense, unable to respond to insulin.

insulin sensitivity   A term that indicates the body's cells respond to insulin correctly. This is the opposite of insulin resistance, in which the body's cells don't respond adequately to insulin and thus don't absorb nutrients, such as blood sugar, efficiently.

ketone bodies   The by-products of fat metabolism. They're made by the liver and are a normal part of metabolism. On a low-carb weight-loss program, the liver makes more ketone bodies than at other times. The amount of ketone bodies produced is indicated on ketone urine strips.

ketosis   The process of making ketone bodies from lipolysis. The ketone bodies are then used for energy. As your body uses its fat for energy, you lose weight.

lipolysis   The breakdown of fat, known as triglycerides, into free fatty acids and glycerol. These fatty acids are then used as energy to fuel the body. Insulin inhibits lipolysis and favors fat storage.

metabolic resistance   A condition in which a person's basal metabolic rate is so low that the person has a difficult time losing weight.

metabolism   The rate at which your body burns fuel. A high metabolism makes it easier for a person to lose weight and keep it off. Having a slow metabolism makes it harder to lose weight. You can increase your metabolism through exercise and by eating the low-glycemic way.

monounsaturated fats   Dietary fats that are highly beneficial to your health and to losing weight. They are typically liquid at room temperature but solidify when refrigerated.

mystery ingredients   Food package ingredients that you can't pronounce are ingredients that you can't easily purchase by themselves at the grocery store (for example, maltodextrins), or are preservatives and artificial colorings. Avoid purchasing products with more than two or three mystery ingredients, if any.

net carbs   The total amount of carbohydrates in a food serving minus dietary fiber and any added sugar alcohols. Net carbs give a good indication of how a food will affect blood sugar levels. Dietary fiber doesn't raise blood sugar levels. Even though sugar alcohol is not a true carbohydrate or a true alcohol, it will raise a person's blood glucose level to a small degree. If you are diabetic, count one half of the sugar alcohol grams as part of your total carbohydrate intake.

nutrient dense   Foods that naturally contain high concentrations of essential nutrients, such as complete protein, essential fatty acids, vitamins, minerals, or antioxidants.

phytonutrients   The nutrients found in plants and plant products, such as vegetables, fruits, nuts, and seeds. Phytonutrients include vitamins, minerals, antioxidants, and glyconutrients.

Pilates An exercise form that originated with Joseph Pilates in the 1940s. It focuses on strengthening the core muscles, which are in the abdominal area. The exercises combine strength training and stretching. The result is long, lean, flexible, and strong muscles, plus great posture.

polyunsaturated fats Dietary fats whose molecules are not "saturated" with hydrogen atoms due to the presence of two or more double carbon bonds. Polyunsaturated fats are liquid at room temperature and remain liquid when refrigerated or frozen.

saccharides The scientific term for sugars. The term includes all sugars, including the sugars we intentionally eat, such as sucrose, fructose, and lactose (the sugar in milk). Saccharides also include other lesser-known sugars present in foods that don't raise blood sugar levels and which are considered non-nutritive because they don't contain calories.

saturated fats A molecular structure that is saturated with hydrogen atoms. Saturated fats are solid at room temperature. Butter and lard are saturated fats.

serotonin A brain neurotransmitter responsible for relaxation and uplifted moods.

stevia with FOS A natural low-calorie and low-carbohydrate sweetener. In its pure state, it's ten times sweeter than sugar with virtually no carbohydrates or calories. Stevia is an herb that originated in South America, and FOSes are fruit ogliosaccharides that nourish the friendly bacteria in the intestines that support gastrointestinal health. Just ¼ teaspoon is equivalent in sweetness to 1 teaspoon of sugar.

toxins Chemical substances that harm or irritate the body. A person can get toxins into the body through breathing, consuming them when eating, drinking, or taking medications, and through skin contact.

trans-fatty acids Fats that are manmade by converting unsaturated vegetable oils into partially hydrogenated vegetable oils through heating, at which time hydrogen atoms become attached to the oils. Partially hydrogenated fats are solids at room temperature and are more chemically stable, meaning that they have a longer shelf life than an unsaturated vegetable oil. Trans-fatty acids have been shown to directly cause clogged arteries and heart disease. They are found in many commercially available baked goods and other processed foods. The FDA requires that all food labels list the amount of trans-fats per serving.

trigger food A food that can lead you to overeating, or even to binge eating. Some common trigger foods are candy, chips, popcorn, donuts, and ice cream. If you have a trigger food and find it impossible to eat only a small amount, it's best not to eat it at all.

Food Listings for Carbohydrates, Glycemic Index, and Glycemic Load

This list includes only information on foods that contain carbohydrates. Animal proteins, such as meats, seafood, and poultry don't contain carbohydrates, so their glycemic index and glycemic load are both zero. The same is true for butter and vegetable oils.

Foods	Glycemic Index Value	Amount	Carbs in Grams	Fiber in Grams	Net Carbs	Glycemic Load
Almond flour	0	1 cup	21	11	10	0
Almonds	0	1 cup	28	15	13	0
Apple juice	40	1 cup	29	0	29	12
Apples	38	1 medium	22	5	17	6
Apples, dried	29	9 rings	37	5	32	9
Applesauce, unsweetened	40	½ cup	13	3	10	6
Apricots	57	3 medium	10	1	9	5

Foods	Glycemic Index Value	Amount	Carbs in Grams	Fiber in Grams	Net Carbs	Glycemic Load
Apricots, dried	30	¼ cup	29	2	27	8
Artichokes	0	½ cup	6	4	2	0
Avocado, California	0	1 medium	12	9	3	0
Banana	52	1 medium	29	4	25	12
Bagel	72	1 small	30	0	30	22
Barley, pearl, uncooked	25	¼ cup	37	6	31	11
Barley, rolled, cooked	66	½ cup	15	2	13	9
Basmati brown rice, cooked	58	½ cup	18	2	16	8
Baked beans	50	½ cup	27	7	11	20
Beets, canned	64	½ cup	6	1	5	3
Black beans, boiled	30	½ cup	20	8	12	4
Black-eyed peas, canned	42	½ cup	16	4	12	5
Bouillon, chicken or beef	0	½ cup	2	0	0	0
Bran, whole wheat	0	2 TB.	5	3	2	0
Brazil nut	0	6 large	4	2	0	0
Bread, 100% whole grain	51	1 slice	13	2	11	7
Bread, white	80	1 slice	15	1	14	11
Bread, whole wheat	77	1 slice	15	1	14	9
Broccoli, raw, chopped	0	½ cup	2	1	1	0
Brown sugar	59	1 oz.	28	0	28	17
Cabbage, raw, shredded	0	½ cup	2	1	1	0
Cantaloup, cubed	65	1 cup	13	2	11	6
Capers	0	1 TB.	1	0	1	0
Carrots, raw, shredded	47	½ cup	6	2	4	3

Foods	Glycemic Index Value	Amount	Carbs in Grams	Fiber in Grams	Net Carbs	Glycemic Load
Cashews	22	¼ cup	8	3	5	3
Cassava	46	½ cup	15	1	14	6
Cauliflower, 1-inch pieces	0	½ cup	3	2	1	0
Celery, diced	0	½ cup	2	1	1	0
Cereals						
All-Bran or Fiber One	30	½ cup	24	14	10	3
Bran Chex	58	½ cup	23	4	19	11
Bran flakes	74	½ cup	22	4	18	13
Cheerios	74	½ cup	11	1	10	7
Cornflakes	92	½ cup	12	1	11	10
Cream of Wheat, cooked	74	½ cup	15	1	14	10
Grapenuts	75	½ cup	31	2	29	22
Oatmeal, instant, cooked	66	½ cup	15	1	14	9
Oatmeal, thick-cut, cooked	53	½ cup	15	2	13	7
Rice Krispies	82	½ cup	11	1	10	8
Shredded Wheat	75	½ cup	15	2	13	10
Cheese, cheddar and Parmesan	0	1 oz.	0	0	0	0
Cherrics, sweet with pits	22	½ cup	12	2	10	2
Chevre cheese	0	1 oz.	1	0	1	0
Chickpeas, canned	42	½ cup	18	7	11	7
Chocolate milk, low-fat	34	1 cup	26	0	26	9
Cocoa powder	55	1 TB.	3	1	2	1
Corn, sweet, boiled	60	½ cup	23	5	18	11
Cornmeal	68	¼ cup	25	3	22	5
Couscous	65	¼ cup	13	2	11	7

continues

Foods	Glycemic Index Value	Amount	Carbs in Grams	Fiber in Grams	Net Carbs	Glycemic Load
Crackers						
Soda crackers	74	6 squares	15	0	15	11
Wheat Thins	67	1 oz.	20	1	19	13
Cream, heavy	0	½ cup	3	0	3	0
Cucumber, sliced	0	½ cup	1.4	1	0	0
Dates	50	¼ cup	32	3	29	15
Donut, cake	76	1 small	23	0	23	17
Eggs, large	0	1 large	0.6	0	0.6	0
Fennel, sliced	0	1 cup	6	2	4	0
Figs, dried	61	3 figs	31	5	26	15
Garlic	0	1 clove	1	0.1	1	0
Grapefruit	25	½ medium	16	6	10	3
Grapefruit juice	48	1 cup	20	0	20	9
Grapes, green	46	¾ cup	19	1	18	8
Green beans, cooked	0	½ cup	5	2	3	0
Green onions	0	¼ cup	2	1	1	0
Green peas, frozen	48	⅔ cup	12	4	8	6
Hazelnuts, diced	0	1 cup	18	7	11	0
Honey, varies widely	55-78	1 TB.	18	0	18	10–20
Ice cream, low fat, vanilla	50	½ cup	9	0	9	5
Jicama	0	½ cup	5	3	2	0
Kidney beans, boiled	46	½ cup	20	7	14	6
Kiwi fruit	58	1 medium	11	3	9	5
Leafy vegetables, raw	0	1 cup	2	1	1	0
Lentils, cooked	29	½ cup	20	8	12	3
Lima beans, frozen	32	½ cup	22	5	17	7
Macadamia nuts	0	¼ cup	5	3	2	0
Mango, sliced	51	½ cup	18	3	15	8
Milk, 2%	32	1 cup	13	0	13	4
Millet, cooked	71	⅔ cup	38	2	36	25

Foods	Glycemic Index Value	Amount	Carbs in Grams	Fiber in Grams	Net Carbs	Glycemic Load
Muesli, no sugar added	54	1 oz.	18	2	16	9
Navy beans, cooked	38	½ cup	36	5	31	12
Oat bran	55	2 TB.	10	5	5	3
Oatmeal, slow cooking, cooked	42	½ cup	13	2	11	5
Orange, sections	42	½ cup	13	2	11	3
Orange juice	53	1 cup	18	0	18	9
Papaya, sliced	56	½ cup	11	3	8	5
Parsnips (cooked)	97	½ cup	13	1	12	12
Pasta						
Spirali pasta (cooked 6 minutes)	43	½ cup	16	1	15	6
Spaghetti (cooked 15 minutes)	64	½ cup	16	1	15	10
Spaghetti (cooked 5 minutes)	38	½ cup	16	1	15	6
Whole-wheat spaghetti (cooked 5 minutes)	32	½ cup	16	2	14	5
Peach, sliced	42	1 cup	14	3	11	5
Peanuts, roasted	14	¼ cup	7	2	5	1
Pear	38	1 medium	25	4	21	4
Peas, frozen	48	½ cup	12	4	8	4
Pecan flour	0	1 cup	15	15	0	0
Pecans, halves	0	¼ cup	5	5	0	0
Pepper, red or green bell, diced	0	¾ cup	4	2	2	0
Pineapple, diced	66	½ cup	19	2	17	8
Pine nuts or piñon nuts	0	¼ cup	5	2	3	0
Pinto beans, canned	45	½ cup	18	6	12	7
Plums, sliced	39	½ cup	11	1	10	5
Popcorn, microwaved	72	1½ cups	14	3	11	8

continues

Foods	Glycemic Index Value	Amount	Carbs in Grams	Fiber in Grams	Net Carbs	Glycemic Load
Potato, white, baked in skin	85	4³/₄ × 2¹/₂ inches	35	5	30	26
Potato chips	57	2 oz.	18	0	18	10
Pretzels	83	1 oz.	20	0	20	16
Prunes, pitted	29	6	34	4	30	9
Pumpkin, cooked	75	1 cup	15	3	12	9
Raisins	64	¹/₄ cup	31	2	29	14
Rice, brown, cooked	50	¹/₄ cup	37	3	35	16
Rice cakes	82	3 cakes	21	0	21	17
Rutabaga, cooked	72	¹/₂ cup	12	2	10	7
Salami	0	1 oz.	0	0	0	0
Soybeans, canned	14	1 cup	19	8	11	2
Split peas, cooked	32	¹/₄ cup	27	11	16	2
Strawberries	40	¹/₂ cup	6	1	5	1
Sucrose, granulated table sugar	68	1 TB.	10	0	10	7
Sweet potato, mashed	44	¹/₂ cup	24	3	21	11
Taco shells, baked	68	2 small	32	2	30	20
Tapioca, cooked with milk	81	³/₄ cup	19	1	18	14
Tomato, chopped	28	1 cup	8	2	6	2
Tortilla chips, plain, salted	63	1 oz.	15	1	14	8
Walnuts, halves	0	¹/₄ cup	3	3	0	0
Wild rice, uncooked	57	¹/₄ cup	34	3	31	18
Yams, cooked, cubed	37	¹/₂ cup	39	3	36	13

Appendix C

Resources

In this appendix you'll find resources that support your glycemic index weight-loss program. Included is information for exercises and supplements, as well as books and websites that will further your knowledge about the glycemic index.

Exercise

Collage Video (www.collagevideo.com)—From yoga to Pilates to kick-boxing, you can find videos on just about any exercise.

Fitballs (www.balldynamics.com)—Improve your core strength, balance, flexibility, and posture by learning how to use resistant exercise balls. This site sells the fitballs and also offers video exercise programs and books.

Anderson, Bob and Jean Anderson. *Stretching*. Bolinas, California: Shelter Publications, 2004. This book teaches you how to improve flexibility and reduce stress while increasing energy through stretching.

Pilates exercise (www.Stottpilates.com)—On this site you'll find information about Pilates exercise as well as videos, equipment, and a listing of instructors in the United States and Canada.

Your local fitness center offers exercise classes, aerobic-training equipment, and strength-training machines. Some have lap-swimming pools, racquetball courts, basketball courts, and tennis courts.

Glycemic Index Lists

www.mendosa.com—The author of this site, David Mendosa, has done a terrific job of building an informative and interesting website that features information on the glycemic index. He includes a complete glycemic index listing of every food tested and includes the glycemic load as well. David also reviews the latest books on the glycemic index and on diabetes.

www.glycemicindex.com—This website is sponsored by the University of Sydney in Australia and contains valuable information on the glycemic index. On this site you can look up the glycemic index of individual carbohydrates. The website contains information from Jennie Brand-Miller, one of the originators of the glycemic index.

Glycemic Index and Glycemic Load Computer Software

GlycoLoad (www.phelpsteam.com/glycoload/)—This downloadable software costs about $16. You'll find listings for all tested carbohydrates. Plus, the program automatically computes the glycemic load of each food based on your serving size.

www.mendosa.com—Print or download a comprehensive glycemic index list with glycemic load for standard-sized servings from this site. Free.

Supplements

- Electrolyte–balancing supplements—Emergen-C electrolyte-balance packets are widely available at grocery and health-food stores. They contain 32 mineral complexes plus plenty of magnesium, potassium, and B vitamins. Mix in hot or cold water and drink. They offer a good energy boost for the late afternoon or after strenuous exercise.

- Greens Plus—Use a tablespoon of this green powder mixed in a glass of water. Contains plenty of antioxidants that will help neutralize your body's acid/ alkaline balance. Helpful for yeast infections and to decrease sugar cravings. Available at www.greensplus.com, www.vitaminshoppe.com, or your local health-food store.

- Fish oil—Take 2 tablespoons per day. Carlson's Fish Oil is lemon-flavored and tastes great. Find at www.vitaminshoppe.com or at your local health-food store.

◆ Psyllium—A fiber supplement that aids in regular elimination and also helps you consume enough fiber daily. Take 1–2 tablespoons in a large glass of water. Then drink one more glass of water. Widely available at health-food stores.

◆ Fennel-seed tea—This is great to lower anxiety and aid in digestion. Steep 1–2 teaspoons of fennel seed in a mug of hot water. Or boil together in the microwave. Available in bulk at health-food stores.

◆ Cortisol-lowering supplements—Following are supplements that will help you lower your levels of cortisol:

    ◆ L-Theanine—This is the soothing component in black or green tea and is widely available at health-food stores in capsule form.

    ◆ B vitamins—Aid in handling stress better. When your body is stressed, it uses them up quickly. Purchase a high-stress B vitamin complex from your health-food store.

    ◆ Liquid B-12—Put a dropper-full under your tongue and you'll find that your stress levels decrease. Widely available at health-food stores.

    ◆ Corterra Xcel—Available at www.nexagenusa.com/bethinpatch. Contains the herbal extracts of hawthorne berries, ashwaganda, and licorice, all excellent to aid you in lowering cortisol levels.

◆ Fat-loss patch—Jen Fe Patch is available at www.Nexagenusa.com/bethinpatch. The healthy ingredients of chromium and Forslean help reduce sugar and starch cravings while normalizing blood sugar levels and supporting the thyroid. Great for aiding in gentle and safe weight loss when combined with low-glycemic eating and frequent exercise.

Appendix D

Sample Menus for Glycemic Index Weight Loss

To help start on your glycemic index weight loss program, here are menu suggestions. You'll find some accompanying recipes in Appendix E.

Body of Knowledge
If you are eating on the Keep It Simple Program, you can modify the menus by omitting the wheat products and instead adding more vegetables—but not white potatoes, which are high glycemic.

Breakfast

Spinach and Red Pepper Egg Omelet

$^1/_2$ cup 100% bran cereal

$^1/_2$ cup skim milk

or

Eggplant Chicken Ricotta

Blueberries ($^3/_4$ cup) with $^1/_2$ cup plain yogurt

or

Cottage Cheese and Tomato Cup

1 TB. peanut butter and 1 slice of coarsely stone-ground whole grain bread

Whole-Wheat Breakfast Burrito

or

Cinnamon and Nut Oatmeal with Berries 'n' Cheese

or

Vegetable Frittata and Fruit

1 cup strawberries

or

Blueberries, Cheese, Nuts, and Cottage Cheese

³/₄ cup fresh or frozen blueberries and 1 small orange sliced

³/₄ cup 2% cottage cheese

2 TB. raw whole almonds

or

Mushroom, Parmesan, Basil, and Tomato Omelet

1 slice of whole-grain pumpernickel toast with 1 tsp. butter

¹/₂ grapefruit

or

Poached Salmon, Fresh Bell Pepper, Fruit

1 cup berries or sliced peaches or pears

Lunch

Grape and Nut Salad with Grilled Chicken

or

Vegetable Medley with Ricotta Cheese and Nuts

or

Homemade Chicken Vegetable Soup

1 large apple or pear

or

Chicken Zucchini with Pine Nuts

$^1/_2$ cup black beans

or

Romaine Lettuce and Beef Wraps

or

Shrimp with Broccoli and Cauliflower

$^1/_3$ cup whole-wheat al dente pasta

or

Chicken, Vegetable, and Bean Salad

or

Grilled Trout, Asparagus, and Winter Squash

or

Romaine lettuce, onion, and tomato salad

Oil and vinegar salad dressing

or

Apple-Walnut Tuna Salad

Dinner

Stuffed Green Pepper with Sirloin

Fresh herbs and onions

2 cups spinach, tomato, onion salad

2 TB. salad dressing (olive oil or canola oil base) of choice (5 grams of carbs or less)

$^1/_3$ cup whole-grain al dente pasta

or

Turkey Breast with Butternut Squash and Spinach Salad

2 cups spinach leaves with onion and olives

2 TB. full-fat salad dressing (olive oil or canola oil base)

or

Cod Fillet with Broccoli and Beet Salad

$^1/_3$ cup basmati brown rice

Endive or Romaine lettuce leaves with $^1/_2$ cup beets (not pickled)

or

Grilled Salmon with Green Beans

Sweet potato or yam

or

Parmesan Chicken with Spaghetti Squash

Lima beans or Edamame

or

Baked Halibut with Artichoke Hearts

Romaine lettuce, onion, and tomato salad

Olive oil and vinegar dressing

Fresh strawberries topped with dab of plain yogurt or whole cream

or

Cornish Hen with Yams and Green Beans

Romaine or spinach, onion, and red pepper salad

Vinegar and olive oil dressing

or

Chicken Stir-Fry with Wild Rice

Snacks

Following is a list of low-glycemic snacks:

- 1 piece of fresh fruit and 12 nuts
- 2 cups vegetables with 1 oz. hard cheese
- 1 cup raw vegetables with $1/4$ cup hummus
- 1–2 cups vegetable soup
- 1 cup winter squash with cinnamon, sprinkled with stevia with FOS
- 1 cup celery sticks with $1/2$ TB. peanut butter
- 2 cups cucumber and onion slices with $1/2$ TB. sour cream or $1/4$ cup avocado dip
- 1 large green pepper and 1 large red pepper, sliced, with 1 oz. cheddar cheese
- 2 TB. cashews and vinegar over 2 cups raw tomato and zucchini slices
- 2 cups vegetable broth soup (nonstarchy veggies) with 1 cup broth and 1 cup veggies)
- 1 cup diced fresh herbs, summer squash, and pea pods with vinegar and $1/2$ cup 2% cottage cheese
- 1 cup snap peas and celery, 1 cup roasted mushrooms, 2 TB. raw whole pumpkin seeds
- 1 cup green cabbage and red pepper coleslaw made with 2 TB. vinegar and oil dressing
- $1/2$ cup Edamame (fresh, green), mixed with 2 TB. almonds wrapped in 3 Romaine lettuce leaves

Recipes

Breakfast

Cottage Cheese and Tomato Cup

Prep time: 5 minutes
Cook time: None
Serves: 1
Serving size: complete recipe

1 cup 2% cottage cheese

2 cups diced tomatoes

$^1/_2$ cup diced cucumber

$^1/_4$ tsp. dried basil

Glycemic index: 25
Glycemic load: 5
Net carbohydrate grams: 18
Fat grams: 4
Protein grams: 31
Calories: 240

Mix cottage cheese, tomatoes, and cucumber with basil.

Saturday Eggs

Prep time: 5 minutes
Cook time: 2 minutes
Serves: 1
Serving size: 2 eggs

2 eggs

1 tsp. butter

$^1/_8$ cup heavy cream

1 TB. shredded cheddar cheese

Glycemic index: 0
Glycemic load: 0
Net carbohydrate grams: 1
Fat grams: 27
Protein grams: 17
Calories: 315

Heat butter in a small skillet over medium-low heat. Gently pour in cream. Crack eggs and pour into pan on top of cream. Gently baste eggs with cream until eggs are cooked through. Sprinkle with cheese and let melt slightly.

Cook's note: Saturday eggs are very rich, so you may find that one egg is plenty. We call them Saturday eggs because they're designed for special days.

Cinnamon Nut Oatmeal with Berries 'n Cream

Prep time: 5 minutes
Cook time: 5 minutes
Serves: 1
Serving size: one recipe

$^1/_4$ cup long-cooking or steel-cut oatmeal

$^1/_2$ tsp. cinnamon

$^1/_2$ tsp. real vanilla extract

2 TB. sliced or whole almonds

$^3/_4$ cup 2% cottage cheese or 2 oz. shredded hard cheese

$^3/_4$ cup fresh berries, such as raspberries, blueberries, strawberries, or blackberries

Glycemic index: 45
Glycemic load: 13
Net carbohydrate grams: 30
Fat grams: 10
Protein grams: 25
Calories: 315

Cook oatmeal with cinnamon per package instructions. Remove from heat. Add vanilla, almonds, and cheese. Stir to mix.

Pour into serving bowl and top with berries.

Vegetable Frittata

Prep time: 10 minutes
Cook time: 5 minutes
Serves: 1
Serving size: 1¹/₂ cups

2 eggs

¹/₄ cup of leftover lean meat or chicken

1 TB. grated Parmesan cheese

1 teaspoon butter

²/₃ cup fresh or leftover vegetables, chopped

¹/₄ cup shredded cheddar or Monterey Jack cheese

Glycemic index: 0
Glycemic load: 0
Net carbohydrate grams: 6
Fat grams: 32
Protein grams: 38
Calories: 555

Beat eggs in a bowl. Add meat or poultry and Parmesan cheese and mix.

Melt butter in a skillet over medium heat. Add vegetables and cook until slightly tender, about 5 minutes. Reduce heat and add egg mixture.

Cover and cook without stirring for about 3 to 5 minutes or until egg is set. Sprinkle shredded cheese over the egg mixture and cover for 1 minute to let cheese melt.

Whole Wheat Breakfast Burrito

Prep time: 10 minutes
Cook time: None
Serves: 1
Serving size: 1 burrito

1 small, low-carb, whole-wheat tortilla

¹/₂ cup diced green pepper

¹/₂ cup diced tomatoes

¹/₄ cup diced onion

¹/₂ cup diced cooked chicken

¹/₄ cup salsa

1 TB. sour cream

Glycemic index: 37
Glycemic load: 7
Net carbohydrate grams: 19
Fat grams: 7
Protein grams: 25
Calories: 295

Combine green pepper, tomatoes, onion, and chicken in small bowl. Stir in salsa. Place whole wheat tortilla on dinner plate. Top with chicken mixture. Fold.

Garnish with sour cream.

Appetizers

Avocado Dip

Prep time: 5 minutes
Cook time: None
Serves: 1
Serving size: 1 recipe

$^1/_2$ fresh avocado

2 TB. fresh lemon or lime juice

$^1/_8$ tsp. cumin

$^1/_8$ tsp. red chili powder

Glycemic index: 0
Glycemic load: 0
Net carbohydrate grams: 2
Fat grams: 17
Protein grams: 2
Calories: 192

Mash avocado into a thick paste. Add lemon or lime juice, cumin, and red chili powder. Mix well.

Sweet Avocado Dip

Prep time: 5 minutes
Cook time: None
Serves: 1
Serving size: 1 recipe

$^1/_2$ fresh avocado

1 TB. fruit preserves or orange marmalade

$^1/_4$ tsp. minced fresh ginger

Glycemic index: 42
Glycemic load: 7
Net carbohydrate grams: 16
Fat grams: 17
Protein grams: 2
Calories: 247

Mash avocado into a thick paste. Stir in preserves and ginger.

Spinach Dip

Prep time: 10 minutes
Cook time: None
Serves: 10
Serving size: $^1/_3$ cup

1 cup fresh or frozen cooked spinach

8 oz. cottage cheese, drained

2 TB. fresh basil, chopped

1 TB. dried dill

$^1/_4$ cup ranch dressing

$1^1/_2$ TB. soy sauce

$^1/_2$ medium onion, chopped

Glycemic index: 24
Glycemic load: < 1
Net carbohydrate grams: 1
Fat grams: $3^1/_2$
Protein grams: 6
Calories: 67

Blend all ingredients in a food processor until smooth. Refrigerate. Serve with cut-up vegetables, such as carrots, broccoli, jicama, snow peas, radishes, or cucumbers.

Turkey or Chicken Quesadillas

Prep time: 30 minutes
Cook time: 4–8 minutes
Serves: 4
Serving size: 1 quesadilla

4 small low-carb flour or corn tortillas

$^1/_2$ cup shredded mozzarella cheese

$^1/_4$ cup shredded cheddar cheese

8 oz. cooked turkey or chicken, sliced

2 green onions, sliced

$^1/_2$ cup finely chopped fresh cilantro

1 tomato, finely chopped, and drained

2 tsp. finely chopped, pickled jalapeño peppers

Glycemic index: 61
Glycemic load: 6
Net carbohydrate grams: 9
Fat grams: 8
Protein grams: 21
Calories: 305

Preheat nonstick skillet over medium heat.

Place tortillas, one at a time, on preheated, nonstick skillet. Evenly distribute 2 TB. mozzarella and cheddar cheeses plus $^1/_4$ chicken, onions, cilantro, tomato, and peppers over top.

Cook over medium heat until cheese melts (tortilla shouldn't brown). Fold to make half-moon; press firmly in place. Transfer to baking sheet or platter in warm oven.

Repeat with remaining tortillas and remaining ingredients.

Cut each into 2 or 3 wedges. Serve immediately.

Chick Pea Dip

Prep time: 10 minutes
Cook time: None
Serves: 6
Serving size: $^1/_3$ cup

2 cups cooked or canned garbanzo beans, drained

1 clove garlic, minced

1 TB. sesame tahini

2 TB. olive oil

1 red pepper, diced

1 TB. lemon juice

$^1/_2$ cup water

Glycemic index: 26
Glycemic load: 4
Net carbohydrate grams: 17
Fat grams: 6
Protein grams: 5
Calories: 106

Blend all ingredients in a food processor or blender. Serve with cut-up vegetables or low-glycemic crackers.

Smoked Salmon Dip

Prep time: 5 minutes
Cook time: None
Serves: 4
Serving size: $^1/_4$ recipe

4 oz. smoked salmon

$^1/_2$ cup sour cream

$^1/_2$ tsp. minced onion

$^1/_8$ tsp. paprika

$^1/_8$ tsp. freshly ground black pepper

Glycemic index: 0
Glycemic load: 0
Net carbohydrate grams: 0
Fat grams: 8
Protein grams: 7
Calories: 125

Cut salmon into small pieces. Place in bowl and add sour cream. Stir to mix. Add onion, paprika, and ground black pepper. Blend well.

Serve with low-glycemic crackers or cut-up vegetables. Or use as a garnish for meat main dishes or salads.

Soups

Gazpacho

Prep time: 20 minutes
Cook time: None
Serves: 6
Serving size: $^3/_4$ cup

2 ripe tomatoes, cut in half

1 small jalapeño pepper, stemmed and seeded

1 clove garlic, peeled

$^1/_3$ cup green pepper, seeded and sliced

1 red bell pepper, seeded and sliced

1 cucumber, cut into 1-inch slices

2 cups V-8 or tomato juice

3 TB. balsamic or red wine vinegar

4 shakes Tabasco sauce, or to taste

3 TB. fresh basil, finely chopped

$2^1/_4$ oz. of sliced ripe black olives (from a can)

1 TB. capers, drained

Glycemic index: 25
Glycemic load: 2
Net carbohydrate grams: 6
Fat grams: 1
Protein grams: 1
Calories: 34

In a food processor, finely chop jalapeño pepper with garlic. Add onion, red and green peppers, and cucumber. Add tomatoes and process. Remove mixture from processor and put into a large bowl.

Stir in V-8 or tomato juice, vinegar, Tabasco, basil, olives, and capers. Chill before serving.

Crab Soup with Bell Pepper

Prep time: 15 minutes
Cook time: 1 hour
Serves: 4
Serving size: $^{1}/_{4}$ recipe

2 TB. olive oil

2 cans crabmeat

2 oz. brandy

2 TB. tomato paste

1 clove garlic, minced

2 quarts water

3 red bell peppers, cut in 1-inch pieces

1$^{1}/_{2}$ TB. minced jalapeño peppers

2 cups sliced fresh mushrooms

2 TB. olive oil

1 bay leaf

6 Roma tomatoes, cut in half

1 large onion, chopped

Glycemic index: 12
Glycemic load: 1
Net carbohydrate grams: 8
Fat grams: 8
Protein grams: 14
Calories: 172

Combine 2 TB. olive oil, crabmeat, brandy, tomato paste, and garlic in water. Bring to a boil and simmer for 30 minutes.

Add peppers, mushrooms, olive oil, bay leaf, tomatoes, and onion. Simmer another 30 minutes.

Avocado Tortilla Soup

Prep time: 15 minutes
Cook time: 20 minutes
Serves: 8
Serving size: 1$^{1}/_{2}$ cups

3 14-oz. cans chicken broth

2 14-oz. cans tomato soup

1 cup diced, cooked chicken

$^{1}/_{2}$ cup chopped cilantro

3 cloves garlic, minced

$^{1}/_{2}$ tsp. chili powder

1 avocado, cut into cubes

8 corn chips, crushed

Glycemic index: 35
Glycemic load: 4
Net carbohydrate grams: 10
Fat grams: 5
Protein grams: 2
Calories: 100

Combine chicken broth, tomato soup, chicken, cilantro, garlic, and chili powder. Bring to a soft boil and simmer for 15 minutes.

Ladle into bowls and top with avocado and crushed corn chips.

Main Dishes

Spinach and Red Pepper Omelet

Prep time: 5 minutes
Cook time: 5 minutes
Serves: 1
Serving size: 1 omelet

1 tsp. butter

2 eggs or 1 egg and 2 egg whites

¼ tsp. chopped basil, fresh or dried

¼ cup diced red pepper

Glycemic index: 0
Glycemic load: 0
Net carbohydrate grams: 1
Fat grams: 10
Protein grams: 14
Calories: 160

Beat eggs lightly with basil in a bowl. Melt butter over medium heat in a small skillet. Add eggs to skillet, cooking until slightly cooked. Add red pepper. Fold omelet in half and cook until set.

Eggplant Chicken

Prep time: 5 minutes
Cook time: 5 minutes
Serves: 1
Serving size: 1 omelet

3 oz. cooked skinless chicken breast, chopped

1 cup fresh eggplant

1 tsp. butter

½ oz. feta cheese

Glycemic index: 0
Glycemic load: 0
Net carbohydrate grams: 5
Fat grams: 8
Protein grams: 22
Calories: 205

Slice and sauté eggplant in one tsp. butter. Add chopped, cooked chicken breast. Stir chicken in with the eggplant mixture and sprinkle with feta cheese. Serve while warm.

Chicken Zucchini with Pine Nuts

Prep time: 10 minutes
Cook time: 10 minutes
Serves: 1
Serving size: 1 recipe

4 oz. skinless chicken breast   1 cup zucchini slices

1 tsp. soy sauce   1 cup tomato slices

2 tsp. olive oil   2 TB. pine nuts

1 tsp. water   Salt and pepper to taste

1 tsp. vinegar

Glycemic index: 15
Glycemic load: 2
Net carbohydrate grams: 10
Fat grams: 15
Protein grams: 32
Calories: 210

In a medium-size skillet, sauté chicken breast in 1 tsp. olive oil. When partially cooked, add soy sauce and water. Cook until done. Slice.

On dinner plate, arrange zucchini and tomato slices. Sprinkle with 1 tsp. vinegar and 1 tsp. olive oil. Sprinkle with salt and pepper to taste. Top with chicken slices. Sprinkle with pine nuts.

Romaine Lettuce and Beef Wraps

Prep time: 10 minutes
Cook time: None
Serves: 1
Serving size: 1 recipe

4 large Romaine lettuce leaves   1 tsp. olive oil

4 oz. cooked lean beef,   ⅓ cup cooked wild rice
cut into strips
                                       4 long toothpicks
2 cups diced tomatoes

2 TB. vinegar

Glycemic index: 39
Glycemic load: 11
Net carbohydrate grams: 26
Fat grams: 14
Protein grams: 30
Calories: 340

Place beef strips, tomatoes, and wild rice in a small bowl and stir in vinegar and olive oil.

Divide mixture evenly among the 4 Romaine leaves. Roll up and secure with toothpicks.

Shrimp with Broccoli and Cauliflower

Prep time: 10 minutes
Cook time: 10 minutes
Serves: 1
Serving size: 1 recipe

¼ cup dry whole wheat pasta

¼ tsp. salt

¼ tsp. olive oil

4 oz. peeled and deveined shrimp

1 tsp. butter

1 cup broccoli

1 cup cauliflower

Glycemic index: 19
Glycemic load: 5
Net carbohydrate grams: 22
Fat grams: 8
Protein grams: 34
Calories: 280

Fill a large saucepan with water. Add salt and olive oil. Heat until boiling. Add pasta and boil 5 to 6 minutes. Drain.

In a covered saucepan, lightly steam broccoli and cauliflower. At the same time, heat butter in a small skillet and then sauté shrimp.

Toss the pasta with shrimp and vegetables.

Grilled Salmon with Green Beans

Prep time: 10 minutes
Cook time: 10 minutes
Serves: 1
Serving size: one recipe

3 oz. salmon, grilled or poached

2 cups fresh green beans, steamed

2 TB. slivered almonds

Glycemic index: 0
Glycemic load: 0
Net carbohydrate grams: 9
Fat grams: 14
Protein grams: 24
Calories: 260

Arrange dinner plate with a base of green beans. Top with salmon. Sprinkle with almonds.

Parmesan Chicken with Spaghetti Squash

Prep time: 5 minutes
Cook time: 15 minutes
Serves: 1
Serving size: 1 recipe

4 oz. skinless chicken breast

1 tsp. soy sauce

2 cups spaghetti squash, cooked

2 TB. shredded Parmesan cheese

$^1/_4$ tsp. dried rosemary

Glycemic index: 0
Glycemic load: 0
Net carbohydrate grams: 15
Fat grams: 9
Protein grams: 31
Calories: 260

Heat water in saucepan to boiling. Add soy sauce and chicken and keep at a gentle boil for about 15 minutes or until chicken is thoroughly cooked. Remove from water and slice.

Toss chicken with spaghetti squash and sprinkle with cheese and crushed rosemary.

Baked Halibut with Artichoke Hearts

Prep time: 5 minutes
Cook time: 5 minutes
Serves: 1
Serving size: 1 recipe

4 oz. halibut

$^1/_2$ cup artichoke hearts

1 TB. vinegar

2 tsp. olive oil

Glycemic index: 0
Glycemic load: 0
Net carbohydrate grams: 5
Fat grams: 13
Protein grams: 29
Calories: 265

Grill or broil halibut. At the same time steam artichoke hearts. On dinner plate, arrange halibut and artichoke hearts. Sprinkle artichoke hearts with vinegar and oil.

Cod Fillets in a Spicy Tomato Sauce

Prep time: 10 minutes
Cook time: 30 minutes
Serves: 8
Serving size: 4 ounces cod plus $1/8$ vegetables and sauce

2 lbs. cod, cut into fillets

$3/4$ tsp. salt

$1/2$ tsp. cayenne pepper or chili powder

$1/4$ tsp. ground turmeric

1 tsp. ground fennel seeds

1 tsp. ground mustard seeds

1 small onion, finely chopped

2 cloves garlic, peeled, finely chopped

1 14-oz. canned, chopped tomatoes

$1/2$ tsp. ground cumin

Glycemic index: 32
Glycemic load: 1
Net carbohydrate grams: 4
Fat grams: 4
Protein grams: 29
Calories: 164

Put all ingredients except cod into a large frying pan. Bring to a boil and simmer gently for 15 minutes. Add fish and simmer for 10 minutes.

Roast Beef, Vegetable, and Bean Salad

Prep time: 10 minutes
Cook time: None
Serves: 1
Serving size: full recipe

3 oz. cooked lean roast beef, cut into strips

2 cups diced celery, cucumber, and carrots

1 cup chopped raw spinach leaves

$2/3$ cup cooked lima beans

3 TB. vinegar and oil salad dressing or

2 TB. regular full-fat, creamy salad dressing

Glycemic index: 23
Glycemic load: 7
Net carbohydrate grams: 28
Fat grams: 16
Protein grams: 23
Calories: 360

In a large salad bowl, layer spinach, vegetables, and beef. Toss with salad dressing.

Apple-Walnut Tuna Salad

Prep time: 10 minutes
Cook time: None
Serves: 4
Serving size: 1/4 recipe

1 6-oz. can tuna

2 TB. mayonnaise

1 large apple, cut in cubes

2 cups diced celery

2 TB. chopped walnuts

Glycemic index: 28
Glycemic load: 3
Net carbohydrate grams: 10
Fat grams: 9
Protein grams: 8
Calories: 163

Combine all ingredients in bowl and mix thoroughly.

Chicken or Pork Stir-Fry

Prep time: 15 minutes
Cook time: 5 minutes
Serves: 1
Serving size: 1 recipe

4 oz. cooked chicken or pork, cut into strips

3 cups combined cut-up green and red peppers, broccoli, water chestnuts, and zucchini, parboiled

2 tsp. canola oil

1/3 cup cooked wild rice

Glycemic index: 25
Glycemic load: 8
Net carbohydrate grams: 30
Fat grams: 18
Protein grams: 33
Calories 402

Using a wok, heat canola oil over medium heat. Add vegetables and stir to coat with oil. Cook 2 minutes. Remove from heat. Place chicken or pork in wok and stir-fry for 1 minute. Return vegetables to wok and stir-fry for 1 more minute.

Serve over wild rice.

Shrimp with Capers

Prep time: 5 minutes, plus 1 hour marinating time
Cook time: 5–10 minutes
Serves: 4
Serving size: 1/4 recipe

2 TB. liquid from jar of capers

2 TB. honey

1 tsp. dried lemon peel or 1 TB. fresh, grated lemon peel

3 TB. lemon juice

1/2 tsp. salt

1 lb. large shrimp, peeled and deveined

3 TB. capers

3 TB. chopped sun-dried tomatoes

2 TB. butter

Glycemic index: 54
Glycemic load: 5
Net carbohydrate grams: 9
Fat grams: 12
Protein grams: 28
Calories: 243

Process liquid, honey, lemon peel, lemon juice, and olive oil in food processor until pureed.

Place shrimp in a bowl and pour marinade over shrimp. Marinate 1 hour.

Heat butter in a skillet over medium heat. Add shrimp, sun-dried tomatoes, and capers and sauté until shrimp are cooked, about 5 to 10 minutes.

Serve garnished with lemon wedges.

Vegetables and Side Dishes

Edamame Salad

Prep time: 20 minutes
Cook time: 5 minutes
Serves: 3
Serving size: 1/3 recipe

1 cup cooked spelt berries or
1 cup cooked wild rice

1 16-oz. bag frozen, shelled
Edamame

1 15-oz. can diced tomatoes or
2 fresh tomatoes, diced

2 cups chopped celery

2 TB. chopped green onions

1 TB. extra-virgin olive oil

1 TB. balsamic vinegar

Salt and pepper to taste

Glycemic index: 21
Glycemic load: 7
Net carbohydrate grams: 32
Fat grams: 14
Protein grams: 21
Calories: 354

Cook Edamame according to package directions. Drain and let cool. In a large bowl, mix all ingredients together. Season lightly with salt and pepper.

Cook's note: You can find spelt berries at the health-food store. Using 1/4 cup of uncooked spelt berries or rice will make 1 cup of cooked berries. Edamame are unprocessed soybeans and are eaten as a vegetable.

Chana Dal with Vegetables

Prep time: 10 minutes
Cook time: 1 to 1 1/2 hours
Serves: 8
Serving size: 1/2 cup

2 cups chana dal

4 cups water

1/2 tsp. fresh minced ginger

1/2 tsp. ground turmeric

1 tsp. cumin seeds

1 small onion, minced

1 TB. minced garlic

1 TB. ground coriander

1 tsp. fenugreek

1/4 tsp. garam masala

1/2 tsp. chili powder

3 cups crushed tomatoes

1/2 tsp. salt or to taste

1 TB. fresh lime juice

Glycemic index: 14
Glycemic load: 3
Net carbohydrate grams: 18
Fat grams: 1
Protein grams: 4
Calories: 74

Put chana dal in a heavy pan along with water. Bring to a boil and remove any surface scum. Add turmeric and ginger. Cover, leaving the lid slightly ajar. Turn heat to low and simmer gently for 1 to 1 1/2 hours or until chana dal is tender. Stir every 5 minutes during the last 30 minutes to prevent sticking.

Stir in the cumin seeds, onion, garlic, coriander, fenugreek, garam masala, and chili powder. Serve.

Cook's note: Chana dal is a legume with a very low-glycemic index. You can leave out the garam masala if you can't find it at your grocery store. The dish is spicy and has an exotic Indian flavor. Serve with green beans, zucchini, or carrot strips.

BBQ Sweet Potato Fries

Prep time: 5 minutes
Cook time: 15–20 minutes
Serves: 8
Serving size: 1/2 potato

4 sweet potatoes (about 8 oz. each), peeled and cut into 1/2-inch wedges

Non-stick cooking spray

1/2 tsp. paprika

1/2 tsp. chili powder

Dash cayenne powder

Glycemic index: 44
Glycemic load: 9
Net carbohydrate grams: 20
Fat grams: 0
Protein grams: 1
Calories: 75

Heat oven broiler to low.

Lightly coat potato slices with cooking spray. Sprinkle sparingly with combined seasonings.

Place in a single layer on broiler pan. Broil for 5 to 10 minutes until lightly browned. Turn and broil other side until lightly browned, about 5 minutes.

Squash Medley

Prep time: 30 minutes
Cook time: 20 minutes
Serves: 6
Serving size: 2/3 cup

3 yellow summer squash, sliced (about 1 1/2 cups)

3 zucchini, sliced (about 1 1/2 cups)

2 medium tomatoes, cut in wedges

1 medium onion, sliced

1/3 cup water

1 1/2 tsp. salt

1/2 tsp. freshly ground pepper

1/4 tsp. garlic powder

1/4 cup fine bread crumbs

1/4 cup shredded Parmesan cheese

Glycemic index: 33
Glycemic load: 3
Net carbohydrate grams: 8
Fat grams: 1
Protein grams: 2
Calories: 57

Preheat oven to 400°F.

Place squash, tomatoes, and onions into a pan with 1/3 cup of water. Add salt, pepper, and garlic powder. Bring to a quick boil. Reduce heat and simmer for about 10 to 12 minutes or until vegetables are tender.

Place vegetable mixture into a 13×9×2–inch glass baking dish. Mix bread crumbs and cheese together and sprinkle over top of vegetables.

Bake at 400°F for 10 to 12 minutes or until bubbly and top is golden.

Grated Carrot and Raisin Salad

Prep time: 10 minutes
Cook time: None
Serves: 2
Serving size: $^1/_2$ recipe

1 medium carrot, grated

2 TB. raisins

$^1/_2$ pear or apple, diced

1 TB. red wine vinegar

2 tsp. olive oil

$^1/_4$ tsp. dried Italian herbs

2 TB. pine nuts

> Glycemic index: 50
> Glycemic load: 9
> Net carbohydrate grams: 17
> Fat grams: 10
> Protein grams: 1
> Calories: 155

Combine grated carrot, raisins, and diced pear or apple. Toss with vinegar, olive oil, and Italian herbs. Sprinkle with pine nuts.

Beet Salad

Prep time: 10 minutes plus 1 hour refrigeration time
Cook time: None
Serves: 4
Serving size: About $^1/_2$ cup vegetables

2 cups canned, sliced beets, drained

$^1/_4$ cup sliced onions

2 TB. red wine vinegar

$^1/_2$ tsp. Dijon mustard

2 TB. olive oil

$^1/_2$ tsp. dried tarragon

Salt and pepper to taste

> Glycemic index: 54
> Glycemic load: 4
> Net carbohydrate grams: 8
> Fat grams: 7$^1/_2$
> Protein grams: 1
> Calories: 90

Combine beets and onions in a bowl.

In a separate bowl, beat together vinegar, mustard, olive oil, tarragon, salt, and pepper.

Pour dressing over beets and onions. Refrigerate for 4 hours before serving.

Feta and Pecan Salad

Prep time: 5 minutes
Cook time: None
Serves: 4
Serving size: about 1 cup

4 cups bite-size pieces Romaine lettuce

2 diced tomatoes

$^1/_8$ cup chopped pecans

$^1/_4$ cup crumbled feta cheese

2 TB. vinegar

2 TB. olive oil

1 tsp. dried tarragon

> Glycemic index: 13
> Glycemic load: 1
> Net carbohydrate grams: 5
> Fat grams: 11
> Protein grams: 3
> Calories: 122

Place lettuce in salad bowl. Add tomatoes, pecans, and feta cheese. Sprinkle with tarragon. Toss with vinegar and oil.

Basil with Mozzarella and Tomatoes

Prep time: 10 minutes
Cook time: None
Serves: 2
Serving size: $^1/_2$ salad

16 basil leaves

8 slices fresh ripe tomato (2 medium tomatoes)

8 slices fresh mozzarella cheese ($^1/_2$ oz. slices)

2 TB. balsamic vinegar

2 tsp. olive oil

> Glycemic index: 28
> Glycemic load: 2
> Net carbohydrate grams: 9
> Fat grams: 15
> Protein grams: 15
> Calories: 225

Arrange 8 basil leaves on each serving plate. Top with 4 slices of tomato and then with 4 slices of mozzarella cheese. Drizzle half the vinegar and half the olive oil onto each plate.

Baked Apples

Prep time: 10 minutes
Cook time: 45 minutes
Serves: 1
Serving size: 1 apple

1 apple, cored	¼ tsp. cinnamon
1 tsp. raisins	Dash nutmeg
1 tsp. honey	Dash ground cloves

Glycemic index: 43
Glycemic load: 13
Net carbohydrate grams: 30
Fat grams: 0
Protein grams: 1
Calories: 130

Preheat oven to 375°F.

Place apple in small baking dish. Fill hollow with raisins. Top with honey, cinnamon, nutmeg, and cloves.

Bake for 45 minutes. Serve hot or cold.

Desserts

Strawberries with Topping

Prep time: 10 minutes
Cook time: None
Serves: 1
Serving size: 1 recipe

1 cup fresh or thawed strawberries

Choice of topping:

- 2 TB. plain yogurt
- 2 TB. heavy cream or whipped cream
- 2 TB. frozen nondairy whipped topping
- 1 TB. chopped nuts

With the plain yogurt and nuts:
Glycemic index: 34
Glycemic load: 4
Net carbohydrate grams: 11
Fat grams: 5
Protein grams: 1
Calories: 85

With the cream and nuts:
Glycemic index: 34
Glycemic load: 3
Net carbohydrate grams: 10
Fat grams: 15
Protein grams: 1
Calories: 175

With the nondairy and nuts:
Glycemic index: 34
Glycemic load: 4
Net carbohydrate grams: 11
Fat grams: 6
Protein grams: 1
Calories: 98

Arrange strawberries in a serving bowl. Top with your choice of topping. Sprinkle with chopped nuts.

Cocoa Crisp Crackers

Prep time: 5 minutes
Cook time: 20 minutes plus 30–40 minutes rest time
Serves: 6
Serving size: $1/6$ recipe

$1/2$ cup unprocessed wheat bran

$1/2$ cup long-cooking oats

1 TB. slivered almonds

1 tsp. vanilla extract

$1/2$ cup egg whites or egg substitute

$1/4$ cup unsweetened cocoa powder

$1/4$ cup Xylitol or 3 TB. powdered stevia

$1/2$ tsp. baking powder

Glycemic index: 48
Glycemic load: 4
Net carbohydrate grams: 9
Fat grams: 1
Protein grams: 3
Calories: 62

Preheat oven to 325°F. Combine ingredients in bowl (mixture will be somewhat dry). Flatten mixture on a cookie sheet. The thinner the spread, the crispier the texture will be.

Bake for 20 minutes. Turn oven off and keep crackers in the oven for an additional 30 to 40 minutes.

Crisp Cinnamon Wheat Bran-Oat Flat Bread

Prep time: 5 minutes
Cook time: 20 minutes plus 30–40 minutes rest time
Serves: 8
Serving size: $1/8$ recipe

$1^2/3$ cup dry unprocessed wheat bran

$1^1/3$ cups dry thick-cut oats

1 cup egg whites or egg substitute

1 TB. cinnamon

1 tsp. baking powder

1 TB. Xylitol or 1 tsp. powered stevia

Glycemic index: 47
Glycemic load: 6
Net carbohydrate grams: 13
Fat grams: < 1
Protein grams: 5
Calories: 86

Preheat oven to 325°F.

Mix all ingredients in a bowl. Flatten dough and press onto a pizza pan. The thinner the spread, the crisper the flat bread.

Bake for 20 minutes. Turn oven off and let bread stay in the oven for an additional 30 to 40 minutes.

Strawberry Frost

Prep time: 5 minutes
Cook time: None
Serves: 2
Serving size: ¹/₂ recipe

2 cups frozen strawberries

1 cup apple juice, frozen into cubes

1 banana (medium)

Glycemic index: 43
Glycemic load: 16
Net carbohydrate grams: 38
Fat grams: 0
Protein grams: 1
Calories: 155

Blend all ingredients in a food processor or blender. Serve in cocktail glasses and eat with spoons.

Hawaiian Shortcake

Prep time: 5 minutes
Cook time: None
Serves: 8
Serving size: ¹/₈ recipe

One recipe Crisp Cinnamon Wheat Bran-Oat Flat Bread

8 oz. light plain cream cheese, softened

2 cups sliced fresh strawberries

1 cup crushed pineapple, drained

Glycemic index: 44
Glycemic load: 4
Net carbohydrate grams: 9
Fat grams: 4
Protein grams: 3
Calories: 92

Spread cream cheese over flat bread. Top with strawberries, then with crushed pineapple.

Chocolate Cookies

Prep time: 15 minutes
Cook time: 20 minutes
Serves: 24
Serving size: 1 cookie

¹/₂ cup butter

¹/₃ cup fructose

1 tsp. molasses

1 egg

¹/₄ cup unsweetened cocoa powder

¹/₂ tsp. vanilla extract

¹/₄ tsp. salt

1³/₄ cups pecan flour (1¹/₂ cups pecan halves processed to a flour in the food processor)

Glycemic index: 23
Glycemic load: 1
Net carbohydrate grams: 4
Fat grams: 9
Protein grams: 1
Calories: 98

Preheat oven to 300°F.

In a mixer, cream butter with fructose and molasses. Beat in egg. Add cocoa powder, vanilla extract, and salt. Slowly stir in pecan flour and mix to a stiff dough.

Form dough into 24 balls and place balls on an ungreased cookie sheet about 1 inch apart. Flatten slightly. Bake for 20 minutes.

Index

salami, 178
sporting events, 208-209
vending machines, 208
soluble fiber, 35-36
South Beach Diet, 279-280
soy products, 129-134
eating tips, 134
glycemic index, 131-132
limitations, 132-133
soy protein isolate, 132
spa-type treatments, reducing stress, 224-225
special event eating tips
business travel, 199-200
festivals, 200-201
holidays
family traditions, 196-197
high-carb foods, 196
low-glycemic foods, 195-196
parties, 197-198
self-control, 194-195
vacations, 198-199
Splenda, 139
sporting events, eating tips, 208-209
stamina and strength training, 253
starches, classification of carbohydrates, 10
start dates, 76
stevia with FOS, 140
stomach, abdominal exercises, 256-257, 266
strength training
abdominal exercises, 256-257
benefits, 250-254
avoid weight-loss sagging, 250
body fat percentages, 252
reducing metabolic resistance, 252
stamina and energy, 253

equipment, 254-255
mechanics, 255
mindfulness, 256
stress, 213
cortisol, 214
cortisol-inducing foods, 216-217
cortisol-reducing supplements, 228-230
management program, 220-222
insulin/stress connection, 22-23, 215-216
reduction techniques
eating tips, 159-160
hot baths, 222
personal pampering, 224-227
stretching, 223-224, 262
sun exposure, 223
stress cycle overview, 214-215
weight-loss
eliminating stress triggers, 218
overview, 217
stretching exercises
abdominal stretches, 266
aches and pains, 261
agility, 262
cortisol connection, 260
equipment, 262-263
illusion of slimness, 262
injury prevention, 262
instructional aids, 264-265
methods, 265
muscle strains, 260-261
stress-reduction, 223-224, 262
timing and location, 264
toxin removal, 261
stress reduction techniques, 159-160
sucralose, 139

sugars
classification of carbohydrates, 10-11
listing of sweeteners, 137-139
saccharides, 17
sun exposure, stress-reduction techniques, 223
super-sized meals, 167
supplements
antioxidants, 16
calcium, 126
cortisol-reducing supplements, 228-230
fats, 152
green drinks, 152-153
guidelines for purchasing, 144-145
usage guidelines, 145
vitamins and minerals, 150-151
calcium, 151
chromium, 151
magnesium, 151
selenium, 151
vanadium, 151
Vitamin B, 150
Vitamin C, 150
Vitamin E, 150-151
warnings, 153-154
weight-loss, 230
sweetened drinks, effects on metabolism, 60
sweeteners, 137-139

T

table sugar, 138
take-along meals, sample menus, 190-192
theanine, cortisol-reducing supplements, 228
"thin" behaviors, modeling, 89-90